D1543690

Perinatal and Neonatal Ethics:
Facing Contemporary Challenges

Kathleen Laganá, RN, PCNS, PhD
Karen Duderstadt, RN, MS, PCNS

Editor
Rita Reis Wieczorek, EdD, RN, PNP, FAAN

Consulting Editors
Margaret Comerford Freda, EdD, RN, CHES, FAAN
Professor, Department of Obstetrics, Gynecology and Women's Health
Albert Einstein College of Medicine
Montefiore Medical Center
Bronx, New York

Kathleen Rice Simpson, PhD, RNC, FAAN
Perinatal Clinical Nurse Specialist
St. John's Mercy Medical Center
St. Louis, Missouri

33-1828-03 12/03
ISBN 086525-097-9

Library of Congress Cataloging-in-Publication Data

Laganá, Kathleen

Perinatal and neonatal ethics : facing contemporary challenges / Kathleen Laganá, Karen Duderstadt ; editor, Rita Reis Wieczorek ; consulting editors, Margaret Comerford Freda, Kathleen Rice Simpson

   p. ; cm.

   Includes bibliographical references

   ISBN 0-86525-097-9

   1. Perinatology—Mo9ral and ethical aspects. 2. Neonatal intensive care—Moral and ethical aspects. 3. Infants (Newborn)—Care—Moral and ethical aspects. I. Duderstadt, Karen. II. Wieczorek, Rita Reis. III. Title

   [DNLM; 1. Perinatal Care—ethics. 2. Ethis, Clinical. 3. Infant Care—ethics—Infant, Newborn.
   WQ 21 L172p 2003]
   RG600.L26 2003
   174'.2—dc21
   2003051187

Published by:
March of Dimes
Education & Health Promotion

Editor
Rita Reis Wieczorek, EdD, RN, PNP, FAAN

Associate Editor
Karen Kroder

Project Manager
Mary Lavan

The mission of the March of Dimes Birth Defects Foundation is to improve the health of babies by preventing birth defects and infant mortality. To achieve this end, the Foundation funds programs of community service, advocacy, research and education. Part of our educational objective includes producing high-quality, low-cost education resources for health care providers, including March of Dimes nursing modules; assessment tools designed to enhance the skills of professionals who work with pregnant women; and videos and brochures to help providers communicate key reproductive health messages to clients.

Some March of Dimes publications may, on occasion, contain controversial views. All such statements and opinions are the sole responsibility of the authors and do not reflect an endorsement by the March of Dimes or the editors unless expressly stated.

To order additional copies of this or any March of Dimes nursing module or to request a free March of Dimes continuing education catalog, call 800-367-6630.

For further information on March of Dimes nursing modules, contact:

   March of Dimes
   Education & Health Promotion
   1275 Mamaroneck Avenue
   White Plains, NY 10605
   Phone: 914-997-4609
   E-mail: profedu@marchofdimes.com
   Web site: marchofdimes.com

TABLE OF CONTENTS

TABLE OF CONTENTS

TABLE OF CONTENTS

Editor Acknowledgements

Special thanks to authors Kathleen Laganá, RN, PCNS, PhD and Karen Duderstadt, RN, MS, CPNP for making their knowledge available to nurses and health care providers through the publication of this module.

We also gratefully acknowledge the following reviewers who so generously shared their expertise:

John E. Collins, MSN, CNM, DrPH(c)
Director, Perinatal Department
Bridgeport Community Health Center
Bridgeport, Connecticut

Kit Devine, MSN, ARNP
Preceptor/Lecturer, University of Louisville School of Nursing
Nurse Practitioner, Fertility and Endocrine Associates
Louisville, Kentucky

Preface

March of Dimes nursing modules provide quality continuing education for nurses who deliver services to mothers and infants in a variety of health care settings. Recent years have seen dramatic changes in the world. All segments of society have been affected, altering our patterns of thinking, our actions and reactions. Technological advances have changed medical and nursing practice. Changing demographics have created new opportunities for providers to serve childbearing families of diverse cultural backgrounds.

The March of Dimes recognizes the need to incorporate new, practical information and theoretical knowledge into nursing practice. To meet this challenge and promote excellent care for mothers and infants, the March of Dimes regularly convenes its Nurse Advisory Council to evaluate the nursing modules, to determine their direction and to recommend development of new titles addressing vital issues confronting nurses today.

General Information

Nursing modules are self-directed learning monographs written by expert nurses for nursing professionals who provide prenatal or perinatal care. Each module addresses a specific topic and provides practical clinical information. Topics range from preconception to the neonatal period and cover changes that occur during the transition from intrauterine to extrauterine life; care of the pregnant woman and her fetus; the labor and delivery period; care of the postpartum woman and her neonate; and current and future critical perinatal health problems. Each module provides background information and caregiving standards to meet these issues and addresses assessment of risk, stabilization of the client and emergency care.

Nursing modules do not supplant didactic educational and clinical experiences. Rather, they provide registered nurses with information to enhance their baseline skills. Differential experiences of the learner may require various levels of guidance to apply the materials to practice; for modules that deal with advanced practice topics, clinical application may initially require close supervision.

Module Format

Each nursing module includes several inter-related components and sections. *Cognitive Objectives* are rooted in the factual nature of each module. *Expected Practice Outcomes* stem from the clinical implications of these facts. *Key Concepts* facilitate identification of major points. The *Pre-/Postinstructional Measurement* assesses learner knowledge of the topic before and after module completion. *Clinical Application* emphasizes and provides reinforcement for clinical aspects of the material and allows transfer and implementation by the learner in a specific clinical setting. *Group Discussion Items* provide additional input from other learners and allow further exploration of cognitive and clinical objectives. *Supplementary Materials* provide annotated descriptions of multimedia resources to further enhance the module topic.

Getting the Most from the Module

To make the best use of a nursing module, learners should first read the *Cognitive Objectives, Expected Practice Outcomes* and *Key Concepts* and then answer and correct the *Pre-/Postinstructional Measurement*. They should then read the module text and proceed to the *Clinical Application*. If the module is used in a group setting, the facilitator will arrange a meeting to discuss the *Clinical Application* and *Group Discussion Items*. As needed, learners should review the *References* and *Supplementary Materials* to reinforce the module content and its utilization in clinical practice. After completing the module, learners can repeat the *Pre-/Postinstructional Measurement* to assess learning.

Evaluation

An evaluation is printed on colored paper and inserted in the module. Participants should remove and complete the evaluation, fold and staple it to reveal the postage-paid portion and post it in a U.S. mailbox. (Note: Group study participants may give the completed evaluation to their facilitator following the study session. Independent study takers may submit the completed evaluation directly to the March of Dimes; see the *Independent Study Application* for instructions.) Ongoing analysis of evaluations provides valuable data that enables the March of Dimes to offer the best possible continuing education for nurses.

Continuing Education Credit

This continuing education activity was approved by the New York State nurses Association, an accredited approver by the American Nurses Credentialing Center's Commission on Accreditation. **It has been approved for 5.22 contact hours for registered nurses.**

American Nurses Credentialing Center/ New York State Nurses Association approval applies only to the nursing education activity and does not indicate approval or endorsement of any commercial product used as part of the activity.

The March of Dimes is also approved as a continuing education provider by the State of California Board of Registered Nursing, Provider #CEP-11444.

This module is also approved for .4 continuing education units (CEUs) for certified nurse-midwives (CNMs) by the American College of Nurse-Midwives (ACNM) (program #2003/085). ACNM approval expires 10/24/05. CNMs should verify the module's approval status at marchofdimes.com/professionals if the module is used after the expiration date.

To qualify for continuing education credit, participants must successfully complete the nursing module via independent study or facilitated group study.

Independent Study
To receive continuing education credit for independent study, each participant must:

1. Be a registered nurse or certified nurse-midwife.
2. Purchase and read the module.
3. Complete the *Independent Study Application* located at the back of the module.
4. Complete the module evaluation (self-mailer).
5. Submit the completed *Independent Study Application* along with the module evaluation to: March of Dimes Nursing Modules, 1275 Mamaroneck Avenue, White Plains, NY 10605

The March of Dimes will notify participants of test results within 8 weeks of receiving the test. Participants with scores of 70 percent or higher will receive a certificate of completion; participants with scores less than 70 percent will be offered a second attempt to pass the test.

Independent study tests and applications are also available on the March of Dimes Web site at marchofdimes.com.

Facilitated Group Study
(Workshop/Grand Rounds/Conference)
A facilitated group study requires facilitation by a qualified registered nurse. A facilitated group study may occur as an in-service edu-

cation program, a workshop or nursing grand rounds or a portion of a larger conference or educational meeting. To receive continuing education credit for facilitated group study, each participant must:

1. Be a registered nurse or certified nurse-midwife.
2. Read the module before the facilitated group study.
3. Participate in the facilitated group study.
4. Provide first and last name and mailing address.

The facilitator must:

1. Be a registered nurse.
2. Arrange time and location for the group study.
3. Facilitate discussion on the content of the module as well as the *Clinical Application* and *Group Discussion Items.*
4. Register as a group study facilitator by sending an e-mail to certificate@marchofdimes.com with name, organization name, mailing address and telephone number.
5. After receiving a confirmation e-mail reply, register the group study and participants and print certificates online at the Nursing Module Certificate Center. The e-mail confirmation will provide the Center's Web address. Required registration information includes module title; study date, location and facilitator; and participant names and addresses.
6. Distribute certificates of completion to participants.

Note: If a nursing module is used as part of a larger conference activity approved for continuing education credit, and continuing education credit is to be awarded for a facilitated group study on the nursing module, use the following formula to calculate the appropriate amount of credit: The number of contact hours/CEUs approved for the conference minus the number of contact hours/CEUs counted for the facilitated group study time plus the number of contact hours/CEUs approved for the module. See the following chart for an example:

Description	Credits
Full-day conference approved for 7 contact hours	7.00
Minus 1 hour for the facilitated group study using *Perinatal and Neonatal Ethics: Facing Contemporary Challenges*	- 1.00
Plus 5.22 hours approved for the facilitated group study on the *Perinatal and Neonatal Ethics: Facing Contemporary Challenges*	+ 5.22
Equals the total number of contact hours awarded for the conference plus the facilitated group study	= 11.22

For additional information, contact March of Dimes Education & Health Promotion at:
  Phone: 914-997-4609
  Fax: 914-997-4501
  E-mail: profedu@marchofdimes.com
  Web site: marchofdimes.com

About This Module

This module addresses contemporary challenges facing nurses who provide care to neonates, childbearing women and their families. The module provides an overview of ethical thought, strategies for identifying and managing moral distress and a holistic case study approach for analyzing ethical dilemmas in the clinical setting. Case studies incorporate three models for ethical decision making.

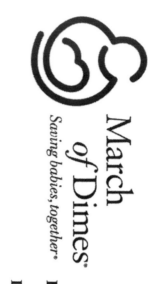

March
of Dimes®

Saving babies, together®

Perinatal and Neonatal Ethics: Facing Contemporary Challenges
Facilitated Group Study Participant Roster

Facilitator _____

Date _____

Location _____

Facilitators may use this sign-in sheet to record participation in the facilitated group study.

	First Name	Last Name	Mailing Address	City	State	ZIP
1						
2						
3						
4						
5						
6						
7						
8						
9						
10						
11						
12						
13						
14						
15						
16						
17						
18						
19						
20						

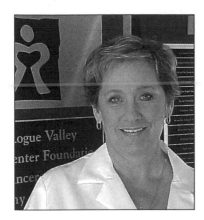

Kathleen Laganá
BS, Oregon Health and Science University School of Nursing, Ashand, Oregon
MS, University of California, San Francisco, California
PhD, University of California, San Francisco, California

Dr. Laganá is a perinatal clinical nurse specialist at Asante Rogue Valley Medical Center Family Birth Center in Medford, Oregon. She is the ethics and legal issues lecturer for Oregon Health and Science University School of Nursing and speaks and writes on the role of advocacy in nursing. She also serves on the ethics comittee at Providence Medford Medical Center in Medford, Oregon. Dr. Laganá designed and wrote the online ethics course for the National Council of State Boards of Nursing. Dr. Laganá began her work in ethics through a March of Dimes grant at the University of California, San Francisco (UCSF) to develop nursing models for ethical decision-making. She studied ethics at UCSF with nursing ethicist Anne Davis.

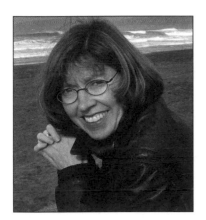

Karen Duderstadt
BS, University of Kansas, Lawrence, Kansas
MS, PNP, University of California, San Francisco, California
PCNS, University of California, San Francisco, California

Ms. Duderstadt is an Associate Clinical Professor in the Department of Family Health Care Nursing at the University of California, San Francisco (UCSF) where she teaches a course on pediatric and neonatal ethical decision-making to graduate students in the pediatric, neonatal and perinatal specialties. She is faculty in the Advance Practice Pediatric Nursing program and supervises students in a variety of clinical settings. She is the former director of Valencia Pediatric Practice, a nurse-managed pediatric primary care practice that provides comprehensive health care to the underserved, multi-cultural population of San Francisco. Ms. Duderstadt is working on her doctorate in nursing at UCSF with an emphasis in health policy.

Upon completion of this module, the learner will be able to:

1. Identify the major systems of ethical thought and the key biomedical ethical principles involved in these systems.

2. Recognize personal morals and values and explore their impact on ethical decision making in the perinatal and neonatal clinical setting.

3. Discuss theories of moral development as they contribute to moral and ethical decision making.

4. Identify the basis of moral distress in contemporary nursing.

5. Describe the role of the nurse in moral advocacy.

6. Recognize the development of the ethic of caring and the role it holds in ethical decision making in nursing.

7. Apply the American Nurses' Association *Code of Ethics for Nurses* in guiding nurses in ethical decision making.

8. Utilize a clinical ethical decision-making model when approaching the resolution of ethical dilemmas.

The learner who meets the objectives and understands the key concepts of this module can be expected to:

1. Participate as an active moral agent in the clinical setting.

2. Uphold the ethical principles in relation to the rights of the fetus, the neonate, the childbearing woman and the family.

3. Take a proactive role in the process of informed consent for the patient and advocate for fetal rights.

4. Support a clinical climate respecting individual differences and diverse cultural and religious beliefs.

5. Support the development of and participate in ethically competent practice in hospital and community agency settings.

The material in this module will help the learner understand the following concepts:

1. The ethical basis for the perinatal dilemma is based on the innate risk of competing rights between the mother and the fetus.

2. Ethical dilemmas exist when there are two conflicting moral principles.

3. A key principle in professional and ethically competent nursing practice is respect for individuals.

4. Ethical dilemma requires the nurse to identify individual morals and values and their effect on clinical decision making.

5. Moral distress for nurses is related to barriers in actualizing the patient advocacy role.

6. Ethical decision making must occur within a holistic social context.

7. A family-centered approach facilitates collaborative decision making and upholds the principles of autonomy.

8. Consensus in an ethical dilemma is best approached via the application of broad ethical decision-making frameworks.

Select the best response to the following questions. Check your answers with the key.

1. Perinatal nurses often experience ethical dilemmas because nurses are:
   A. *Care givers*
   B. *Maternalistic*
   C. *Nonjudgmental*
   D. *Patient advocates*

2. When assisting patients to make decisions that involve ethical dilemmas, nurses must first:
   A. *Refrain from imposing their values on patients*
   B. *Clarify their values in relation to the moral issues*
   C. *Understand ethical theories and principles before making decisions*
   D. *Elicit the thoughts and feelings of the patient and significant others*

3. When information is presented so that a patient can make an informed decision, the health care provider's teaching is based on the principle of:
   A. *Justice*
   B. *Respect*
   C. *Veracity*
   D. *Nonmalfeasance*

4. From the deontologic point of view, the parental decision to withhold neonatal intensive care for a very-low-birthweight infant violates the principle of:
   A. *Utility*
   B. *Justice*
   C. *Autonomy*
   D. *Happiness*

5. Which statement best reflects ethical thoughts from the school of utilitarianism?
   A. *Individuals have a right to make their own decisions.*
   B. *Sanctity of life takes precedence over quality of life.*
   C. *The result of the decision promotes the greatest benefit for society.*
   D. *The decision adheres to regulations that guide moral reasoning.*

6. An ethic of caring exists when a nurse:
   A. *Has values similar to those of the patient*
   B. *Expresses sympathy for a fetus that is to be aborted*
   C. *Makes moral judgments specific to each patient situation*
   D. *Focuses on care that supports the fetus rather than the mother*

7. In ethics, the phenomenon known as "the slippery slope" means that:
   A. *Adherence to ethical principles can gradually erode.*
   B. *Rules change depending on the patient's socioeconomic status.*
   C. *Moral values slip and slide because they are dynamic rather than static.*
   D. *The decision-making continuum begins with paternalism and ends with autonomy.*

8. When considering theories of moral development in relation to women, Kohlberg's theory is to role expectation as Gilligan's theory is to:
   A. *Caring*
   B. *Curing*
   C. *Loving*
   D. *Knowing*

9. Which technological advance most threatens the concept of social justice and could precipitate moral distress for a nurse?
   A. *In vitro fertilization (IVF)*
   B. *Zygote intrafallopian transfer (ZIFT)*
   C. *Gamete intrafallopian transfer (GIFT)*
   D. *Preimplantation genetic diagnosis (PGD)*

10. In health care, the primary, universal, motivating, ethical principle in the provision of care is the obligation to:
    A. *Do good*
    B. *Tell the truth*
    C. *Distribute care evenly*
    D. *Treat people as individuals*

11. The American Nurses Association *Code of Ethics for Nurses* provides guidelines for professional practice because nurses:
    A. *Are able to be more objective than patients*
    B. *Need to encourage good decisions by patients*
    C. *Sometimes need to make decisions for patients*
    D. *Have an obligation to preserve the interests of patients*

12. The first step when using any ethical decision-making model in perinatal nursing is:
    A. *Exploring parental wishes*
    B. *Identifying possible actions*
    C. *Calculating potential outcomes*
    D. *Determining the nature of the problem*

13. A public health objective in *Healthy People 2010* is to eliminate health disparities. This objective is related directly to the ethical concept of:
    A. *Justice*
    B. *Fidelity*
    C. *Veracity*
    D. *Nonmalfeasance*

14. The ethical concept of autonomy was fully upheld in the outcome of:
    A. *Roe vs. Wade*
    B. *The Baby Doe case*
    C. *The Baby Theresa case*
    D. *Buzzancas vs. Buzzancas*

Answers to Pre-/Postinstructional Measurement

1.D 2.B 3.C 4.B 5.C 6.C 7.A 8.A 9.D 10.A 11.D 12.D 13.A 14.B

autonomy—the right to self-determination; the right and responsibility of the competent individual to make decisions about the rightness or wrongness of his/her actions or beliefs

beneficence—the obligation to do good

deontology—ethical school of thought that relies on professional duty to make decisions

dilemma—a difficult choice between unsatisfactory alternatives (Davis & Aroskar, 1983)

ethical act—an act directed toward and that affects another individual (Loewy, 1996)

ethical dilemma—a choice that has potential to violate ethical principles

ethics—a discipline that deals with right and wrong and with moral duty and obligation; comes from the Greek word "ethos," meaning customs or character

fidelity—the obligation to keep promises

justice—equal or comparative treatment of individuals

moral—relating to principals of right and wrong; comes from the Latin word "mores," meaning custom, manners or habit; often considered synonymous with ethical

moral agent—one who makes and acts on a moral decision (Thompson & Thompson, 1985)

moral dilemma—a difficult choice between alternatives that are both right and good and where no one supreme principle presents obviously to determine moral choice (Beauchamp & Childress, 1994)

moralist—one who engages in reflection and discussion about what is right or wrong and guides moral judgment

nonmalfeasance—the obligation to do no harm

paternalism—a system under which an authority makes decisions for others

personification of the fetus—the belief that, as a developing human being (even though unborn), the fetus holds claim to the rights provided to all members of society

practical dilemma—a difficult choice, but one that does not produce a moral dilemma

respect for persons—recognition of individualism and connection to the broader community; recognizes the obligation or duty to others, as well as to self, in making decisions

surrogate decision-maker—individual who makes decisions for someone who lacks the capacity for autonomous choice (i.e., a neonate)

utilitarianism—ethical school of thought that actions are right if they produce consequences of happiness or the absence of pain; striving to bring about the most good for the most people

utility—the greatest good to an individual; an action that is valued

veracity—the obligation to tell the truth; informed consent is an example of adherence to veracity

Perinatal and Neonatal Ethics: Facing Contemporary Challenges

A unique aspect of the perinatal ethical dilemma is that perinatal nurses advocate for two individuals—the woman and the fetus.

Kathleen Laganá
Karen Duderstadt

Perinatal Ethical Dilemma

A dilemma is a difficult choice between unsatisfactory alternatives (Davis & Aroskar, 1983). An ethical dilemma is a choice that has potential to violate ethical principles. The essence of the ethical dilemma in nursing is often based on the nurse's commitment to patient advocacy. A unique aspect of the perinatal ethical dilemma is that perinatal nurses advocate for two individuals—the woman and the fetus. A frequently encountered perinatal dilemma is one in which the mother's legal and ethical right to self-determination (autonomous choice) conflicts with the health care provider's plan of care for the fetus. For example, a pregnant woman experiencing preterm labor desires discharge home to a remote area, while her provider feels that proximity to a neonatal intensive care unit (NICU) is needed to protect the immature fetus if delivery ensues. Should the mother's autonomy be upheld with a discharge plan, or should the decision be based on what is best for the fetus? Strong ethical arguments exist for both actions; however, both actions violate either the rights of the mother or the rights of the fetus.

Ethical arguments in perinatal health care are further complicated by the legal definition that the fetus is not an autonomous individual—it is legally incompetent and not able to independently make health care decisions. Inability to practice self-determination creates a state of vulnerability for the fetus and, in civil societies, calls for protection. Regardless of legal definition, however, some may consider a fetus to be an individual.

Figure 1 illustrates the ascendancy of fetal rights. Based on the 1970 Roe v. Wade decision, personal rights of the

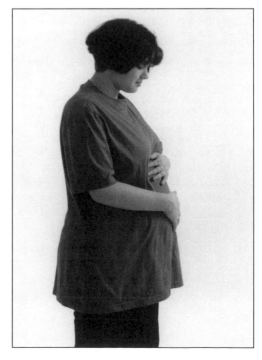

Autonomy upholds the right and responsibility of a competent individual to make decisions about the rightness or wrongness of his/her own actions or beliefs.

fetus theoretically increase at the age of viability (Francoeur, 1983). As the non-competent fetus takes on greater degrees of personhood, social responsibility to protect the fetus also increases, to the point that society might perceive the fetus' need for protection as greater than the woman's need for protection or her right to self-determination under the law. The perinatal nurse's advocacy role is more clearly assigned for the pregnant woman than for the fetus. As maternal and fetal needs are more clearly seen as interdependent, nurses face an ethical dilemma in perinatal care. Efforts to facilitate moral actions may frustrate the nurse advocate within the current financial and political constraints in health care.

Overview of Ethical Thought

Socrates (469-399 B.C.) established the science of ethics, and modern health care ethics are based on the works of Socrates, Plato (428-347 B.C.) and Aristotle (384-322 B.C.). Socrates believed that individuals should never do what is morally wrong, but should maintain a higher moral ground and adhere to what is right, regardless of consequences or what others will think. He argued that reason, rather than emotion, should determine ethical decisions (Frankena, 1973). If this is the basis for ethical decision mak-

ing, then the perinatal nurse must have a clear mind and factual information to act as a moral agent. A moral agent is one who makes and acts on a moral decision (Thompson & Thompson, 1985). Nurses are legally and morally responsible for their actions, and, therefore, directly or indirectly, are moral agents. Nurses must also support and sustain patients who face hard moral choices. Complex ethical situations in the health care arena go beyond the traditional rules of conduct; therefore, it is imperative that health care decisions be based on knowledge of ethical rules and principles.

Ethical Principles

Socrates established basic principles from which ethical thought is derived. These principles serve as guides for ethical actions and are the foundation for ethical philosophies. Socrates acknowledged that sometimes two or more principles apply to the same case but do not lead to the same conclusion.

Autonomy

Autonomy is the right to self-determination. Autonomy upholds the right and responsibility of a competent individual to make decisions about the rightness or wrongness of his/her own actions or beliefs. The principle of autonomy is protected by the U.S.

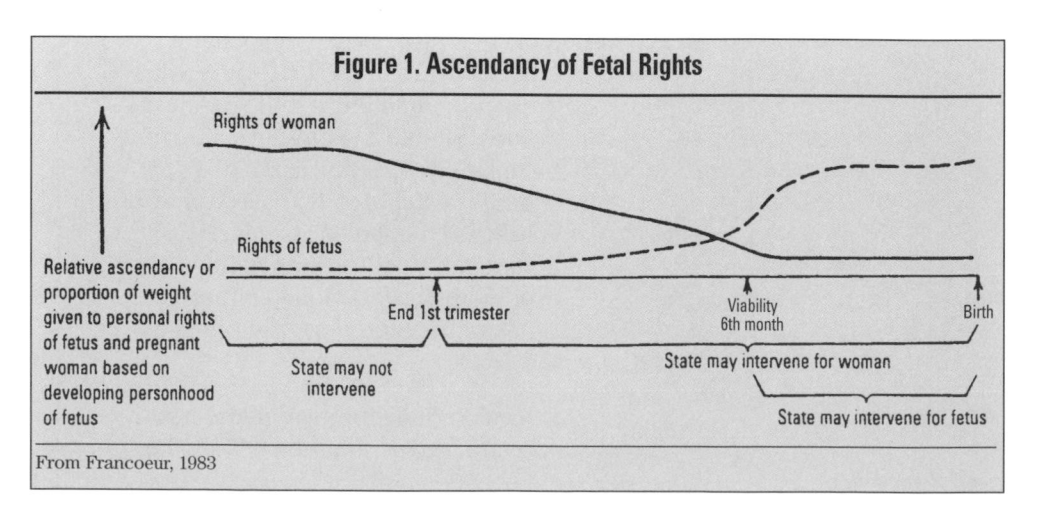

Figure 1. Ascendancy of Fetal Rights

Rights of woman

Rights of fetus

Relative ascendancy or proportion of weight given to personal rights of fetus and pregnant woman based on developing personhood of fetus

End 1st trimester

Viability
6th month

Birth

State may not intervene

State may intervene for woman

State may intervene for fetus

From Francoeur, 1983

Constitution and federal law and is upheld by many professional position statements. The right to autonomous choice is rarely challenged in overt ways.

Based on competency, there are three types of individuals who lack the capacity for autonomous choice: the unconscious person, the individual lacking mental ability to make decisions and the very young, such as the neonate. Parents or other assigned surrogate decision-makers are required for children until emancipation at 18 years of age, with some exceptions. Adolescents who become pregnant are emancipated in most states in relation to their reproductive rights and can determine the outcome of their pregnancies. Pregnant women admitted for perinatal services determine some aspects of autonomous choice by Advance Directives, which are initiatives that act as a kind of informed consent for future interventions in the event that one loses decision-making capacity. The Patient Self-Determination Act of 1990 (42 U.S.C. sec. 1396a) legalized the use of Advance Directives, and they are required for all women in labor and delivery units.

Respect for Others
According to this principle, all persons are equally valued. It includes not only adherence to the principle of autonomy, but also the recognition of individual rights within the context of the broader community or society. Respect for others is a key component in the American Nurses Association's (ANA) *Code of Ethics for Nurses with Interpretive Statements* (ANA, 2001) (Appendix 1).

Beneficence
Beneficence is the obligation to do good. In perinatal health care, health maintenance and prevention of complications uphold this principle. For ex-

ample, when health care professionals treat patients, they are upholding the principle of beneficence. Supporting a low-birthweight infant medically until that infant is physiologically stable upholds the principle of beneficence, as does comforting a family who has experienced perinatal loss. Beneficence in health care depends, to a large extent, upon a health care provider's knowledge of treatment efficacy and the context of the patient's environment.

Nonmalfeasance
Closely associated with the principle of beneficence is nonmalfeasance, the obligation to do no harm. Upholding the principle of nonmalfeasance is a challenge to perinatal and neonatal health care providers, largely due to the power of technology to sustain life coupled with the inability to see the future. Long-term outcome for the individual patient is never known; therefore, decision making is often dependent on health outcome statistics. At times, in the nurse's efforts to do good, harm does occur. The principle of nonmalfeasance asks that the dilemma between the possibility of good outcomes and the risk of poor outcomes always be considered.

Justice
Justice is the principle of equal or comparative treatment of individuals. This principle asks that persons be treated fairly. Justice seeks to distribute benefits and burdens equally throughout society. The principle of justice emphasizes individual rights and equality in moral relationships.

Fidelity
Fidelity refers to faithfulness or the obligation to keep promises. It is a moral obligation and a social virtue. The rule of fidelity guides the actions of an individual in principles of veracity, privacy and confidentiality.

Justice is the principle of equal or comparative treatment of individuals.

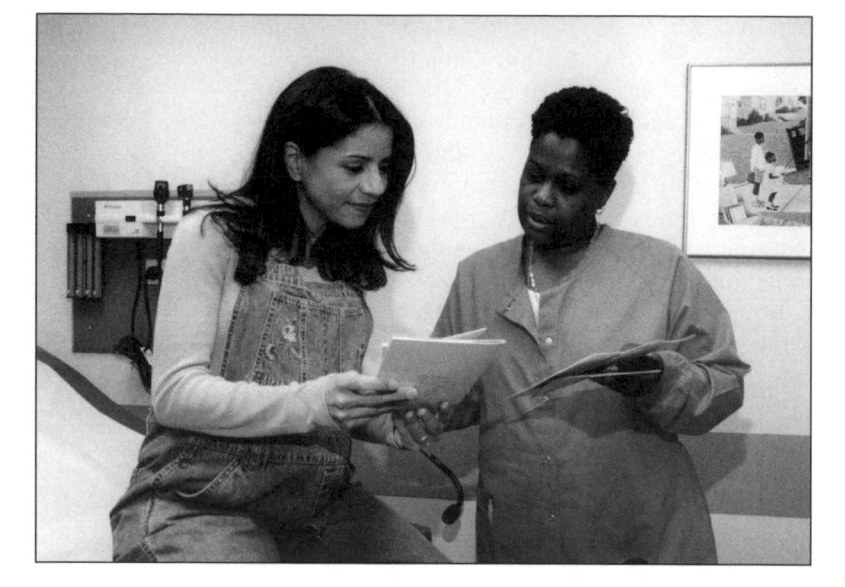

Veracity

Veracity is the obligation to tell the truth. Along with autonomy and respect for others, veracity forms the basis of informed consent in health care. It is closely associated with the principle of fidelity, in that health care providers enter into a contract with clients to provide care and to protect the client from foreseeable harm. To do so, the provider must disclose the risks and benefits of the proposed care.

In some cases, veracity could contribute to harm, representing a classic dilemma of opposing ethical principles. For example, following full informed consent, a client may decline a recommended intervention. An example is the recommended practice of inducing labor to prevent fetal and neonatal infection for women with ruptured membranes. A discussion of the risks of oxytocin might lead the pregnant woman to decline this intervention, putting herself and the fetus at risk for infection. Her right to autonomy, combined with her right to informed choice, may override other considerations.

Utility

Utility is viewed in terms of the greatest good to an individual or an action that is valued. The worth of an individual or action can be judged in different ways. The goal of the principle of utility is to find the single greatest good to balance the interest of all persons affected.

Ethical Dilemma

Although nursing has a professional code of ethics, nurses often face ethical dilemmas. What should I do? What harm or benefit will result from this decision or action? A dilemma is created by conflicting rules and moral principles (Beauchamp & Childress, 1994). Often, the right decision may not necessarily be a good decision for all involved. Perinatal nurses often need moral justification for their decisions that provides sufficient grounds for belief and action.

Conflicts between self-interest and moral requirements often produce practical dilemmas. A practical dilemma presents difficult questions and oral perplexity but does not produce a moral dilemma. Moral dilemmas exist when different approaches or actions are supported by differing ethical principles. Moral dilemmas require developing and assessing one's beliefs to reach a decision.

Nurses are often faced with practical dilemma. For example, multiple tasks and responsibilities present a dilemma when two clients need assistance at the same time. The nurse must decide which client to assist first. It becomes a moral dilemma when the rights of an individual are challenged by two competing actions. An example of a moral dilemma is the need to use interventions with associated side effects, such as induction of labor with oxytocin. Oxytocin has associated risks, including the rare uterine rupture. The principle of beneficence (to do good by promoting active labor) competes with nonmalfeasance (to do no harm).

Ethical Philosophies

Virtue Ethics

Socrates, Plato and Aristotle argued that distinctions of moral character include the cardinal virtues of courage, temperance, wisdom and justice (Pence, 2000). Human society functions best with virtue ethics. Virtue ethics balances the application of ethical principles and permits moral growth. The framework of virtue ethics introduces character and morality into principle-based ethics and focuses on the virtuous person, rather than on obligations and rights.

Virtue ethics can be a guidepost for a moral life, but defining what is "good" can be difficult. If community welfare is the basis of all human endeavors, then virtue ethics supports an effective framework for decision making. If, as Aristotle claimed, a virtuous person strives for balance by applying rules and principles, then virtues and rules shape each other and permit moral growth (Loewy, 1996). Virtue ethics provide the basis for moral decision making in society and establishes a framework for all ethical philosophies.

Virtue ethics has limitations as it relies on the intrinsic good of an individual and does not guide the individual in how to make moral choices. Therefore, it is an ethical ideal, rather than a practical guide, and is not applied as part of the ethical decision-making model in nursing.

Deontology

Duty comes from the Greek word *deonteis*. In deontology or duty ethics, nurses do not consult their feelings about what to do; instead, they reflect upon their professional duty. In deontology, specific rules guide moral rea-

soning. For example, it is good or right to tell the truth. It is wrong to tell a lie or take the life of another. The emphasis is on motive and not on consequences. This theory relies on the work of Immanuel Kant (1724-1804), who believed rules and principles set for an individual should be universal to all, and that it is one's duty to adhere to them. Kantian ethics (duty ethics) has had a profound effect on modern medical ethics. He believed in the power of humans to use reason to solve their problems.

In deontology, an individual's moral values are of major significance. When an individual makes a moral decision, that moral decision stands in any similar dilemma. However, principles sometimes conflict and do not assist the moral agent in resolving a situation. For example, if the nurse tells the truth, even though the truth will undoubtedly harm the patient, the principle of veracity, or telling the truth, conflicts with the principle of nonmalfeasance, to do no harm.

Utilitarianism

Deontological ethics provides a framework within which decisions about specific problems and concrete situations can be made, but it gives little direction to solving problems of social justice that form an important part of medical ethics (Loewy, 1996). When it comes to questions of allocating health care resources, utilitarian ethics seems more appropriate.

The moral foundation of utility, the "greatest happiness principle," is that actions are right if they produce consequences of happiness or the absence of pain (Mill, 1987). Happiness is good. Promoting the absence of pain is beneficence. In a social order driven by utilitarian morality, the action that brings the greatest good to the greatest number of people would be the moral-

In deontology or duty ethics, nurses do not consult their feelings about what to do; instead, they reflect upon their professional duty.

Table 1. Ethical Arguments in Utilitarianism	
Argument	**Description**
Allocation of resources vs. cost effectiveness	Relates to distribution of scarce health care resources
Quality of life vs. sanctity of life	Addresses the question of preservation of life at all costs
Withholding vs. initiating treatment	Relates to the delivery of care to individuals; questions when care should be initiated, withheld or withdrawn
Paternalism vs. autonomy	Addresses the question of who should make decisions about health care delivery

ly most defensible action. It is the utilitarian perspective that has led to the idea of health care systems that offer the best possible outcomes to the greatest numbers of people. Some refer to this as health care rationing. The utilitarian asks, "Where best may scarce health care dollars be spent?"

The classical origins of the utilitarian theory come from the writings of Jeremy Bentham (1748-1832) and John Stuart Mill (1806-1873). Utilitarians believe that individuals always should produce the maximum balance of positive value in their actions and that the right act is the one that produces the best overall result in a given circumstance (Beauchamp & Childress, 1994). Bentham and Mill conceived of the principle of utilitarianism as an action bringing the greatest good or the greatest happiness. The goal is to choose between alternative courses of action to provide the greatest collective happiness or, if that fails, the least unhappiness. Frankena (1973) further interpreted this system of thought as looking at actions and rules in terms of what the consequences would be for the general welfare if everyone acted similarly in a given situation. Consequences to be considered good must achieve the greatest good for the greatest number (Loewy, 1996). Table

1 identifies ethical arguments in utilitarianism.

Utilitarians often distinguish between the consequences of general acts in particular circumstances and the general rules that determine which acts are right and wrong (Pence, 2000). Act-utilitarianism asks, "What good and bad consequences will result from this action in such circumstances?" In contrast, for the rule-utilitarian, an act must conform to a moral rule or principle, and that conformity makes the act right (Beauchamp & Childress, 1994). Inherent conflict exists between these two interpretations. If the fundamental principle of utility is to maximize the value of an action, then adhering to a particular rule may not prove the most beneficial to the persons affected by the action.

Western society strongly values the principle of autonomy. From a utilitarian perspective, however, there may be times when paternalism is justified. Paternalism is a system under which an authority makes decisions for others. This dilemma addresses the question of who should make decisions about the delivery of health care to individuals, including decisions regarding when care should be initiated, withheld or withdrawn. Often paternalists view their knowledge and judgment superior to the individual's, and individuals may not be fully aware of treatment options or long-term outcomes. Public health policy laws that limit access to care for certain interventions are generally developed by health care experts, informed citizens and lawmakers for the well-being of citizens, thus enacting an ethical principle that Plato called rational paternalism (Bandman & Bandman, 1995).

Justice is also often considered in utilitarian terms. A just society seeks distributive justice by distributing resources equally to all its members. The idea of a social contract is based in the early works of Plato; he argued that human beings cannot survive alone, and that the social nature of human beings requires individuals to form agreements about how to live together (Plato, 1998). Ethicist Thomas Hobbes (1599-1679) argued in support of the social contract, stating that if people were left alone to serve their own self-centered means, there would be no social order (Bandman & Bandman, 1995).

Justice can be seen as a balance between competing claims, for example, in competition for health care dollars. Justice, as a social ideal, asks society to consider the responsibility for social cooperation and an assignment of rights and duties to its members (Rawls, 1999). The prevalent argument is that, in a just society, optimal health is a right.

Despite limitations, strengths exist in utilitarianism for the formation of public policy. The principle demands a just social distribution of health care resources and promotes a goal of social welfare. Utilitarians evaluate the consequences of a society where what affects one does not, in some way, affect all. The goal is that action balances the maximum interest of all affected persons. Utilitarianism is reflected in recent public policy health care decisions, such as the Children's Health Insurance Program, established in 1997, that extends health insurance to large numbers of uninsured children in the United States.

Ethic of Caring

Moral reasoning in the ethic of caring involves empathy and concern and emphasizes responsibility in relationships with others (Carse, 1991). The care orientation rejects impartiality as a moral point of view and understands moral judgments as situation-specific and attuned to particular relationships. This orientation is not specific to gender or discipline, but correlates with an orientation of those who believe that care is dominant and takes precedence in approaching moral problems (Gilligan, 1982). In principle-based ethics, the principles rule without exception to context or relationship. An important role for moral principles exists in care ethics, but care ethics moves away from principle-driven moral judgment.

The ethic of caring is not a complete theory; rather, it is a methodological approach that holds caring as the central concept of ethical decision-making. For many, the problem with the ethic of caring is that caring does not make people moral. The ethic of caring supports the concept that nurses should care and that caring is a moral quality. What is explicit in this approach is that nurses should care about the right things in the right way and encourage what is morally important (Allmark, 1995).

Perinatal and Neonatal Ethics

Perinatal and neonatal ethics have always been driven by the idea that pregnant women and neonates are vulnerable members of society and are

Perinatal and neonatal ethics have always been driven by the idea that pregnant women and neonates are vulnerable members of society and are not always able to defend their rights.

The concept of fetal rights is at the heart of many discussions of perinatal ethics.

not always able to defend their rights. Patient advocacy provides for that defense. However, unique to the field of perinatology is the idea that, during pregnancy, there are two patients for whom health care providers advocate. Historically, conflict has occurred between the rights of the mother and those of the fetus.

Recent rulings have shown a marked increase in respect for maternal autonomy. Court-ordered cesarean section deliveries and perinatal interventions against a woman's choice have been declared brutish and unethical, changing the climate of perinatal care (ACOG, 1987b). Family-centered care, while the accepted standard, is bringing patients and families into collaborative decision making with health care providers. What once was seen as maternal/fetal conflict is often more correctly a case of maternal/provider conflict and resolvable through patient education and respectful communication (Macklin, 1995; Ryan, 1990).

While the issue of opposing rights continues to present in the clinical setting, the nature of perinatal ethical dilemma is evolving into one of challenges in upholding the principle of social justice and the right to health care. Health care costs, growing numbers of uninsured families, increasing population diversity, a shortage of registered nurses and increasing demand for technology all challenge the provision of ethically sound health care. To address social justice, health care providers must examine ethical issues from the perspective of the daily lives of patients.

The nature of ethical dilemmas experienced by nurses is changing. Content on ethics has become standard, entry-level nursing education. Many state nurse practice acts require enactment of the patient advocacy role, usually in the form of providing for patient safety

(ANA, 2001). Better educated and more articulate about ethical practice, nurses may find themselves questioning not the right or wrong of a situation, but how they can facilitate the right.

Maternal/Fetal Conflict

In discussions of maternal/fetal conflict, the mother and fetus are often cast as adversaries (Hornstra, 1998). The concept of fetal rights is at the heart of many discussions of perinatal ethics. Technology has allowed the visualization of the fetus' sucking, swallowing and breathing movements. Gender is easily detected. Baby memento books hold early ultrasound images of the fetal face or toes. It is easy to note how human-like the fetus is at a very early gestation. Personification of the fetus is the belief that as a developing human being (even though unborn), the fetus holds claim to the rights provided to all members of society.

Personification of the fetus is not a contemporary concept. Hippocrates believed that human beings were "preformed" in male semen. Figure 2 depicts this imagined, preformed human called Homun Culus (Meyer, 1939). With the development of primitive microscopy in the 1600s, scientists reported actual visualization of preformed humans in semen (Francoeur, 1985). Today, technology allows a remarkable view of intrauterine life and strengthens the argument for fetal rights, especially when the fetus is near the age of viability.

The foundation for argument concerning the extent of fetal rights lies in the absence of an operational definition of what determines personhood. When does personhood begin? At conception? When the fetal heart begins to beat? When cerebral brain activity is evident? At birth? Or later? Is an immature fetus, unable to survive

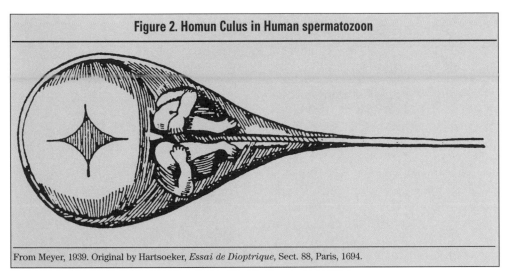

Figure 2. Homun Culus in Human spermatozoon

From Meyer, 1939. Original by Hartsoeker, *Essai de Dioptrique*, Sect. 88, Paris, 1694.

without the bodily support of its mother, an individual person or a physical extension of its mother? Fletcher (1979) presented the concept of the error of potentiality, wherein "that which has potential for being" is at times confused with "that which is." Francoeur (1985) believed that the concept of humanization of the fetus cannot be seen as personhood, as it does not address the human spirit, which encompasses cerebral functioning and the development of human values and beliefs.

Mamatoto is a Swahili word that describes the inseparable nature of the maternal/baby union (Dunham, 1991). Ancient wisdom, as well as current cultures, speak to the importance of maternal health and well-being during pregnancy. However, with the availability of technology to directly aid the fetus, the holistic nature of the maternal/fetal unit has unraveled. Modern perinatal technology has not been the global panacea that it was once hoped. Rising rates of premature birth (U.S. Department of Health and Human Services [DHHS], 2001) continue to be the norm in the industrialized world where perinatal technology is accessible to pregnant women. Today, the health care industry possesses technology to visualize, monitor, surgically repair and eliminate a developing fetus. If the fetus has a degree of moral claim as an individual, then providers must consider that individual's right to health care or, perhaps more fundamentally, the right to life. Whatever the moral obligation owed to the fetus, the U.S. Supreme Court decision Roe v. Wade (1973) clearly stated that after the age of viability, the fetus has enough of a hold on individual rights to deserve protection under the law. The decision upheld a woman's right to pregnancy termination but placed limits on the practice of abortion by introducing the idea of considering the rights and protection of viable fetuses.

Neonatal Rights

Society views beginning of life issues differently than end-of-life issues. The innocence and potential of the newborn evoke different considerations and judgements than do advanced age and frailness of the elderly. As with end-of-life issues, technology has affected neonatal rights. Until recently, most fragile neonates of very low birthweight succumbed to congenital defects or to overwhelming septic

The health care provider must consider clinical decision making based on rational compassion, the values of the persons involved and the cultural context.

infections. Technology has made many neonatal health conditions treatable, but underlying issues exist in salvaging all viable neonates (Loewy, 1996).

The health care provider must consider clinical decision making based on rational compassion, the values of the persons involved and the cultural context. Quality of life is fundamental to clinical ethical decisions regarding the neonate and may warrant further regulatory protection by society. Decisions involving the rights of the neonate may be as difficult, ir not more so, than those involving the fetus.

Surrogate Decision-Makers

All patients, including neonates, who lack the capacity for autonomous choice require a surrogate decision-maker. Surrogate decision-makers are persons close to the patient and who know the patient best (Loewy, 1996). For neonates, surrogate decision-makers are most often parents or members of the health care team. The surrogate decision-maker sets aside his or her own interest and makes decisions based on the patient's best interest, taking into consideration the patient's culture and specific medical situation.

Health care professionals, as well as parents, are moral agents who must have the freedom to act within their own moral boundaries and cannot be forced to violate their own ethical beliefs or superimpose their beliefs on others (Loewy, 1996). However, surrogate decisions may conflict with societal norms and ethical principles, as evidenced by the 1982 Baby Doe case.

Baby Doe

Baby Doe was born April 9, 1982 at Bloomington Hospital in Indiana. He was diagnosed with esophageal atresia and Down's syndrome. His parents, after conferring with physicians, legal counsel and hospital administrators,

chose not to consent to surgical repair of the esophageal atresia and asked that the infant not receive nutrition or fluids and be allowed to die. The hospital unsuccessfully attempted to obtain a court order from local and state courts to treat the infant, and prosecutors began work on an appeal to the U.S. Supreme Court. Baby Doe died six days after birth.

The Baby Doe case created a public and political furor resulting in the Baby Doe Rule, Public Law 98-457. The law stated that physicians must treat all infants with life-threatening conditions unless, in the physician's responsible medical judgment, the infant is chronically or irreversibly comatose; unless the treatment would prolong dying or is futile in terms of the survival of the infant; or unless the treatment would be not only futile but inhumane (*Federal Register*, 1985). The Baby Doe regulations defined medical neglect to include withholding of medically indicated treatment from a handicapped infant with a life-threatening condition. The law equated withholding potentially life-saving treatments with homicide, child abuse and neglect (Moreno, 1987). The appellate court eventually ruled the Baby Doe regulations invalid. However, the issue of whether and under what circumstances medical treatment and medical support should be withheld from critically ill infants remains highly volatile, and subsequent legal rulings have provided no single answer (Vernon, 1998).

The ethical principles of beneficence and nonmalfeasance are at odds with the Baby Doe regulations. Courts generally question medical decisions when parents wish to withhold or terminate medical treatment (Vernon, 1998). However, courts have upheld parental rights to determine the extent of medical treatment for their infant as long as it does not constitute abuse or

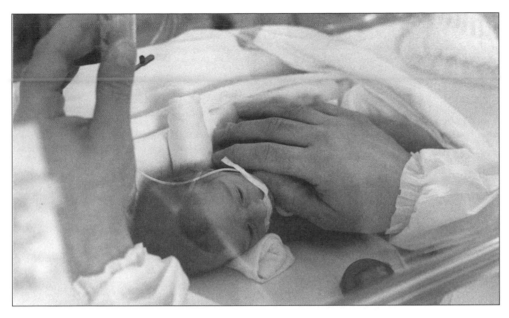

neglect. The Baby Doe case pitted sanctity of life against quality of life and questioned a parent's right to choose one over the other for a child. For many, the right to life holds a stronger moral obligation than a parent's right to decide. In the aftermath of the Baby Doe case, neonatologists found that the original ruling did not allow adequate consideration of infant suffering in deciding whether to initiate or discontinue life support (Kopelman, Irons & Kopelman, 1988).

Science Dominating Human Life

Much of the political and legal maneuvering so evident from the Baby Doe case camouflaged a deeper ethical concern—the growing dominance of medicine and science over human life. The risk of paternalism is great in neonatology because of technological advances and enthusiasm for life-sustaining treatments. The use of perinatal and neonatal technology and the enthusiasm generated in the media by its success have made the work of health care providers very public. More than ever, consumer expectations drive decision making. Vimpani (1991) identified the "technological imperative"—

because we have the technology, we must use it. What is the moral responsibility of health care providers to patients and society? Should resources needed for health promotion and for combating societal inequities be sacrificed for technological advances? Is it necessary to draw lines of constraint around perinatal and neonatal health policy? Health care providers struggle to give some moral direction to these ongoing debates.

Often medical and nursing staff must balance life-support measures with quality of life and medical futility. Quality of life considerations frequently emerge in cases of non-treatment or cessation of treatment. Prolonging life with treatment that gives no reasonable chance of relieving suffering, or that leads to suffering without the hope of recovery, is unethical. Furthermore, the prognosis for an impaired neonate has implications for the family's quality of life (Pence, 2000). Caring for a severely handicapped child imposes enormous burdens on the family. By extending the lives of severely damaged or underdeveloped neonates, are the medical and nursing professions causing more harm than good? Since the Baby Doe case, a more flexible legal standard has emerged. State laws now consider quality of life and medical futility in medical ethical decision making and generally base legislation on parental authority (Doroshow et al., 2000).

In a review of clinical decision making in the NICU, Wall and Partridge (1997) found that medical futility determined medical decisions more frequently than quality of life in cases where death was imminent, or when medical interventions only prolonged the suffering of a marginally viable neonate. Medical futility was documented in 74 percent of cases of neonates who died from withdrawal of life-sustaining treatments; quality of life issues were indicated in only 23 percent of the cases. Death by withdrawal or withholding life support is more common in NICUs than death that occurs during use of maximal support (Wall & Partridge, 1997).

Access and availability of neonatal intensive care has increased the number of infants who receive aggressive treatments; however, these treatments are often later determined to be inappropriate (Wall & Partridge, 1997). Providing treatment regardless of outcome is increasingly under question. Should the fair distribution of resources affect ethical considerations in treatment options? Cost-benefit analysis is being applied to what is technologically possible. Providing treatment of doubtful value regardless of cost is clearly not mandated (Doroshow et al., 2000).

The earlier and more vigorously nurses participate in decision making around initiation and maintenance of life-support, the greater the consensus among staff in a unit. Hazebroek and colleagues (1996) found that infants had a higher risk of mortality in NICUs

where staff attitudes differed about infant care plans. Most often, nursing staff disagreed over care of neonates who were not receiving full life support. Anticipated poor quality of life may have played a role in the judgments of health care team members. The findings in this study speak to the importance of team decision making in NICUs around initiation or maintenance of life support and probable quality of life. Detecting and discussing provider attitudes may improve overall medical outcomes and benefit the working environment.

Negotiation and Practice

Ethics committees or consultants often function in a step approach, first thinking of theory, then analyzing principles to be applied and, finally, individualizing the approach to a particular case (Loewy, 1995). However, in actual practice, nurses, other health care team members and ethics consultants act as negotiators. Loewy (1995) likens the practice of ethics for the negotiator to an approach often used by travel agents. In arranging travel, agents ask three questions: Where are we now? Where do we want to go? How do we get from where we are now to where we want to go? Often in health care delivery, providers determine where they are with a case without asking the other important questions—where do they want to go and how do they get there? This can lead to dissension and confusion in the health care team. Disagreement about medical facts is a technical problem, not a moral dilemma, and is resolvable by expert consultation.

The negotiator allows patients and families to come to an agreement with health care providers by analyzing the context of the problem, presenting alternatives and identifying important distinctions and possible outcomes (Loewy, 1995). This process, if given time, usually comes to a successful conclusion. Throughout this process, ethical theory, ethical principles and care ethics must work together toward a common goal.

Values and Moral Development

Health care professionals must resolve ethical dilemmas before taking deliberate action. On a personal level, all individuals hold values based on their culture, religion, family upbringing and general education. One of the most difficult aspects of socialization into a profession is accepting the professed values of that profession. Nurses face two kinds of dilemmas. The first is the internal dilemma where they must face their own beliefs and reconcile them to determine their moral view (Loewy, 1996). Each nurse's moral view is shaped by personal experience. The second dilemma is external, in which nurses must reconcile their own points of view with that of their patients, their patients' families, other members of the health care team and legal demands. The external dilemma often occurs when nurses make assumptions about patients. Assumptions create conflicts and misunderstandings. Professionals must reconcile the moral process of internal dilemmas and justify the process and conclusions of external dilemmas to produce consensus and understanding (Loewy, 1996).

Value Clarification

Value clarification is a dynamic process that fosters the nurse's understanding of self. Even though public affirmation of values is important, nurses do not have the right to impose their values on others. Clarifying personal values and understanding ethical principles and theories facilitate systematic ethical decision making and foster moral development. The nurse as a moral agent has a professional responsibility to protect and defend the ethically based rights of patients. Moral agents must act and assume responsibility for that action. Understanding ethical thought provides the nurse with a systematic way of approaching personal and professional ethical decision making.

Theories of Moral Development

Moral reasoning is the mental process that intervenes between recognition of a moral dilemma and the reaction to a moral dilemma. It is the decision-making process by which the nurse chooses among personal moral values to appropriately respond to a moral dilemma.

Kohlberg's Theory

Much of the current nursing literature utilizes Kohlberg's theory of moral development (Table 2). Kohlberg's conceptual framework presents three distinct levels of moral reasoning and subdivides each level of morality into two stages. Each stage of moral reasoning represents a distinct moral philosophy, with implications for an individual's moral orientation to society. For example, Kohlberg felt that women often operate at the mutual morality level of moral reasoning by doing what society expects of them. To move beyond this stage requires women to see beyond the relationships that bind their moral experiences (Kohlberg, 1984; Omery, 1989). Kohlberg's ultimate concern is with morality itself (Allmark, 1995), and many nursing theorists criticize Kohlberg's framework because it fails to recognize the uniqueness of women's moral and relational social perspective.

Gilligan's Theory

Gilligan (1982) interpreted the stages of moral development differently (Table 3). He argued that feminine moral reasoning is simply different from masculine moral reasoning because women have developed a sense of responsibility based on the universal principle of caring. Gilligan's moral concept of care is consistently reinforced as an ideal by those who serve the needs of others. Gilligan's work, along with that of Noddings, Benner and others, forms the basis for the ethic of caring applied to the nursing profession (Held, 1995).

Advocacy and Moral Distress

Nurses are moral agents because they are in a position to act for the welfare of others (Laganá, 2000). Nurses generally spend more time with patients than do other health care providers, and they often develop caring relationships with patients. This relationship is sometimes referred to as "knowing the patient" (Laganá, 1994; Tanner, Benner, Chesla & Gordon, 1993) and includes an understanding of the patient's perspective and experience, leading to empathy and concern. From a professional perspective, caring and patient

Table 2. Kohlberg's Theory of Moral Development	
Level I: Preconventional morality	Stage 1: Heteronomous morality—Right is equal with authority.
	Stage 2: Instrumental authority—Right is what is fair.
Level II: Conventional morality	Stage 3: Mutual morality—Right is doing what is expected of people in your role.
	Stage 4: Social system morality—Doing right is meeting the actual duties of your role.
Level III: Postconventional or principle morality	Stage 5: Social contract morality—Right is doing the greatest good for the greatest number.
	Stage 6: Universal ethical morality—Right is following the universal ethical principle of justice.

Adapted from Omery, 1989

Table 3. Gilligan's Model of Moral Development
Level I: Orientation to individual survival Transition: From selfishness to responsibility
Level II: Goodness as self-sacrifice Transition: From goodness to truth
Level III: Morality of nonviolence Nonviolence becomes the moral guide governing all moral reasoning; care is the universal obligation.

Adapted from Gilligan, 1982

advocacy are responsibilities. However, at the interpersonal level, the motivation for advocacy is naturally greater when a caring relationship exists.

Moral distress involves a fundamental conflict with the nurse's professional value system and the inability to act in a given moral dilemma. Learning to identify moral conflict and finding the strength to carry out moral resolves are part of the process of moral work

that is critical for the integrity of nursing (Tiedje, 2000). Tiedje (2000) presents a model that reflects the cognitive, behavioral and emotional dimensions of the moral process (Figure 3). It involves moving from an initial, morally confronting situation through moral decision making, moral distress and, finally, moral action. The model recognizes that learning to identify moral conflict is critical to the difficult process of carrying out moral work.

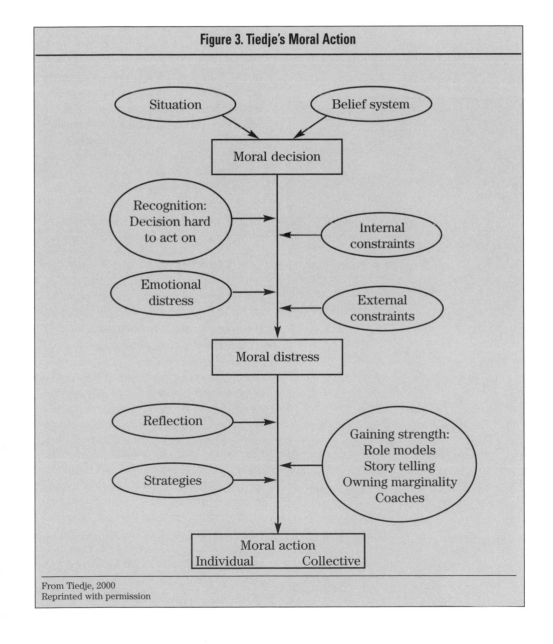

Figure 3. Tiedje's Moral Action

From Tiedje, 2000
Reprinted with permission

How does the nurse assume the role of moral agent? The extent to which the nurse should act is controversial. It is often necessary to take risks that go beyond questions of moral principles and values. Generally, nurses can make moral decisions about particular cases, but Jameson (1993) recognized that nurses experience moral distress when they are unable to carry out their moral decisions.

Nurses maintain a unique position between the patient and the bureaucracy of the health care system; however, they often lack the power to act for their patients. Nurses often experi-

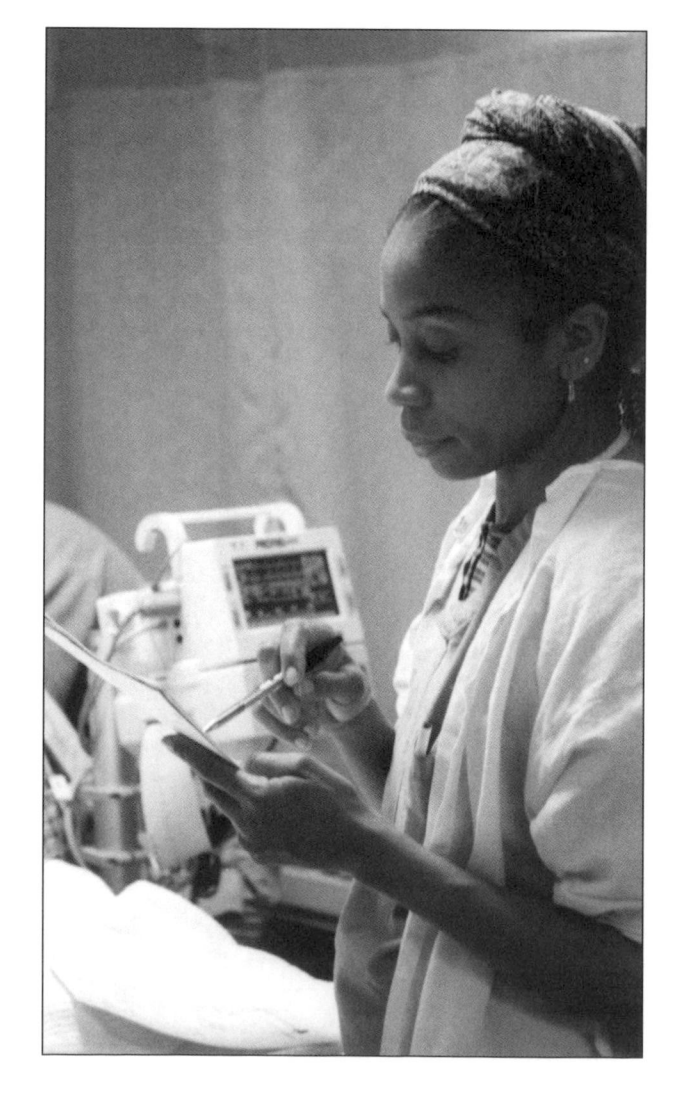

ence moral distress when obligations to employers and patients are at odds (Tiedje, 2000). Caffrey & Caffrey (1994) noted that the ethic of caring in nursing often conflicts with the health care system's value for fiscal solvency. Increased fiscal demands on the health care system under managed care have made the nurse's role as patient advocate more difficult, and nurses often are unable to act on their moral decisions.

Moving Toward Moral Action

To move to moral action, nurses must devise effective strategies in the health care setting that are respectful and honest (Andre, 1998). Nurses have the advantage of working within systems while, at the same time, holding professional autonomy. This provides a unique opportunity for promoting change. To do so, nurses must move to positions of empowerment within the system. Nursing leadership must promote professional autonomy, clinical excellence and nursing participation on ethics committees, departmental committees, professional organizations and in legislative activities.

Advocacy requires the use of power (Falk Rafael, 1996). "Whistle blower" laws may provide nurses with legal support when they must move beyond system limitations or expose ethical violations, such as denial of fair and legal access to care, breach of confidentiality or denial of a patient's autonomous choice.

Cameron (1981) identified the risk of disconnection between what is known to be right and the actions that actually occur. Nurses must believe they can make a difference and will be able to bring about change for their patients. Nurses can draw on the collective strength of shared experiences to move beyond moral distress to moral action (Wilkinson, 1987-1988).

Code of Ethics for Nurses

Professional codes guide members in moral action, professional accountability and responsibility by providing guidelines without dictating behavior (Rumbold, 1999). Codes must be sufficiently broad to be universally accepted by a profession's members. The American Nurses Association's (2001) *Code of Ethics for Nurses with Interpretive Statements* addresses the profession's obligation to respect human dignity, to uphold the fidelity of the professional relationship and to advocate for the patient. It also calls for improving the nursing work environment and promoting the profession's role in building health care systems that meet the public's needs. Professional values, when incorporated into the individual nurse's value system, become a standard for behavior in clinical practice.

The *Code of Ethics for Nurses* provides a guide for professional behavior. It is limited, however, in assisting the process of ethical decision making. The Code's provisions and interpretive statements do not provide criteria for ethical decision making in nursing practice or a systematic framework for ethical decision making. Knowledge of ethical principles and rules is needed to provide direction for ethical nursing practice (Gaul, 1989). The nurse as a moral agent must continually assess the ongoing dynamics of clinical situations and assist other moral agents, such as family members or physicians, in proposing alternatives and making decisions.

Contemporary Challenges in Perinatal and Neonatal Ethics

Perinatal Outcomes and the *Healthy People 2010* Objectives

Healthy People 2010 is the latest installment in a series of national health objectives that began in 1979 as a report from the U.S. Surgeon General on health promotion and disease prevention (U.S. Department of Health, Education and Welfare, 1979). *Healthy People 2010* objectives subscribe to the ethical principle of distributive justice. The first of the original *Healthy People 2010* goals was "to continue to improve infant health and, by 1990, to reduce infant mortality by at least 35 percent, to fewer than 9 deaths per 1,000 live births" (U.S. DHHS, 2000, p. 21). From the perspective of social justice, "No cold statistic expresses more eloquently the difference between a society of sufficiency and a society of deprivation than the infant mortality rate" (Newland, 1982, p. 321). Infant mortality transcends politics or worldview (Laganá, 1996) and is a point of national embarrassment in the United States. Morally, failure to protect the most vulnerable members of our society represents a break in the social contract. The United States continues to lose rank internationally in this area, despite an enormous financial expenditure in the treatment of premature infants.

Healthy People 2000 (U.S. DHHS, 1990) set more specific objectives for decreasing the infant mortality rate, decreasing the number of low-birthweight infants and increasing access to prenatal care. While the United States came close to reaching its goal of a 7 percent infant mortality rate (7.2 percent), as of 1995, the United States continued to lag behind nearly all other industrialized nations. Furthermore, other critical measures of increased risk for infant mortality (such as low birthweight and prematurity) have increased (U.S. DHHS, 2000).

Public health objectives in *Healthy People 2010* are based on two overarching goals: to increase the quality and years of healthy life and to eliminate health disparities. Health disparities

From a public health perspective, the most challenging problem facing perinatal health care providers is the failure of perinatal interventions to reverse the trend of premature birth.

generally are perceived as a failure to equally distribute resources. When these disparities are associated with gender, race or ethnicity, the concern becomes more urgent. A major focus of *Healthy People 2010* is maternal, infant and child health. Twenty-three objectives address the following areas: 1) reduction of fetal, infant and child deaths; 2) reduction of maternal death and illness; 3) improved prenatal care; 4) improvements in obstetric care; 5) reduction of risk factors, including substance use; 6) reduction of birth defects; and 7) improved newborn care, including breastfeeding, newborn screening and health care services (U.S. DHHS, 2000).

In an affluent society like the United States, it is difficult to justify or understand why infant mortality and poor birth outcomes continue to be public health problems. Because medical technology has done little to prevent the complex socioeconomic problems that contribute to poor health outcomes, national health policy recognizes the need for an increased focus on creating healthy communities. This is a public health model. As the nation addresses the *Healthy People 2010* objectives and public funds are expended to work toward these goals, questions of utility are raised. Resources must be spent on treating existing health problems (such as prematurity) unless society as a whole decides not to treat these problems. Perinatal technology has been instrumental in improving maternal and infant health outcomes once complications arise. However, costs associated with this technology are monumental. The utilitarian might argue that prevention is less costly than expensive technological treatments and should hold priority status.

Perinatal Technology, Diagnosis and Research

Patients expect health care providers to use safe and proven methods. Providers must advise patients of treatment risks and knowledge limits. From a principle-based ethical perspective, fidelity becomes an issue when providers fail to address limitations or validity of research studies with patients. Patients enter into a trust relationship with health care providers based on an agreement that the provider will advocate for the patient's best interests.

Efforts to improve maternal and fetal well-being are grounded in the ethical principle of beneficence. Perinatal technological advancement primarily has been in the area of perinatal diagnosis, such as obstetrical ultrasound, electronic fetal monitoring and amniocentesis. While these technologies have advanced to the point of allowing rare, in-utero correction of fetal problems, such as diaphragmatic hernia or blood dyscrasia, prevention of many perinatal problems remains elusive. From a public health perspective, the most challenging problem facing perinatal health care providers is the failure of perinatal interventions to reverse the trend of premature birth.

The Ethical Challenge of Preventing Prematurity

An ethical concern arises when expenditures for health care do not result in improved outcomes. The principle of fidelity, the obligation to keep promises, is violated when interventions do not cause intended good health outcomes. Management of preterm labor is an example. Low birthweight (LBW) (<2,500 g) is a major indicator of infant morbidity and mortality (Shiono & Behrman, 1995; U.S. DHHS, 2001) and requires costly health care services (Lewit, Baker, Corman & Shiono,

1995). While a small number of full-term infants are born LBW in the United States, LBW more often affects infants born prematurely (before the 37th week of gestation). Seventy-five percent of infant mortality and 50 percent of long-term neurological morbidity in the United States is due to preterm birth. Preterm labor is the most common reason for hospitalization during the antenatal period (Agency for Health Care Research and Quality [AHRQ], 2000). The March of Dimes nursing module *Preterm Labor: Prevention and Nursing Management*, 3rd Edition (Freda & Patterson, 2004) provides a nursing overview of preterm labor.

The United States has been relatively successful in decreasing its infant mortality rate; however, preterm labor presents a more complicated picture. While statistics on the incidence of preterm labor are not available, the rate of preterm birth in the United States is clearly documented. Between 1990 and 2000, the rate of preterm births increased by more than 9 percent (March of Dimes, 2002a). The 2000 preterm birth rate of 11.6 percent was over 50 percent higher than the *Healthy People 2010* objectives of 7.6 percent (March of Dimes, 2002a). Preterm births of multiple-gestation infants influenced this rate only slightly (Centers for Disease Control and Prevention [CDC], 2000b).

An analysis of singleton preterm births provides a surprising picture of ethnic and racial disparity. Preterm births for non-Hispanic Blacks are nearly twice that of non-Hispanic Whites; however, between 1989 and 1996, preterm births for non-Hispanic Blacks actually decreased by 9.9 percent (CDC, 1999b). Other ethnic and racial minorities, while less extreme, demonstrated similar trends. Surprisingly, non-Hispanic

Whites experienced an 8 percent increase in preterm births (CDC, 1999b); the reason for this increase is poorly understood. An examination of gestational age at birth for all population groups shows that 76.5 percent of singleton births in the general population occurred between 33 and 36 weeks gestation (CDC, 1999b). It is important to explore how improved care, such as patient education or regionalization, has influenced preterm birth.

Although babies born between 33 and 36 weeks gestation are at risk of serious complications, including respiratory distress syndrome and other prematurity-related problems, they are less likely to die than infants born at earlier gestational ages; therefore, they are protected by the principle of justice and a universal right to life. Ethical issues concerning the principle of justice also arise from the racial and ethnic disparity in preterm birth in the United States. Where racial and ethnic disparity exists, society must question the equitable distribution of social resources.

Preterm labor intervention has undergone close scrutiny. Based on the principle of veracity, an important part of informed consent is the knowledge of risks and benefits in any medical intervention. Despite active management of preterm labor over the last few decades, the rate of preterm births in the United States has increased (Lam, 1991; CDC, 1999b). The treatment of preterm labor commonly includes intravenous hydration, bedrest, prophylactic antibiotics and administration of tocolytic drugs with intermittent or continuous uterine activity monitoring. To avoid cervical change, preterm labor contractions are treated early with tocolytic drugs that may not be necessary (Flynn, 1999). Pharmaceutical drug classes most commonly used in the treatment of

The March of Dimes Prematurity Campaign will invest $75 million over 5 years and will raise new funds to support research into the causes and treatment of prematurity.

preterm labor are betamimetics (terbutaline and ritodrine), magnesium sulfate, calcium channel blockers (nifedipine) and prostaglandin inhibitors (indomethacin) (Flynn, 1999).

Efforts to prevent preterm delivery have associated risks that require the application of nonmalfeasance. Preterm labor management, especially tocolysis, is associated with maternal complications, including gastrointestinal disturbances, metabolic problems, muscular weakness, pulmonary and cardiovascular complications and affective mood problems, such as anxiety and depression (AHRQ, 2000; Flynn, 1999). Additionally, evidence exists that some treatments for preterm labor lead to poor fetal outcomes. An example is the practice of administering multiple courses of antenatal corticosteroids during preterm labor to speed fetal lung maturity. A review of the literature suggests that multiple courses of corticosteroids may contribute to reductions in neonatal head circumference and increased rates of low birthweight and maternal and neonatal infection (Walfisch, Hallak & Mazor, 2001). Antenatal indomethacin administration is associated with neonatal complications, including patent ductus arteriosus, gastrointestinal complications, oligohydramnios and increased risk for intracranial hemorrhage (Norton, Merrill, Cooper, Kuller & Clyman, 1993).

The principle of veracity requires that providers disclose the effectiveness of treatments as part of the informed consent process. The use of first-line tocolytics, such as betamimetics and magnesium sulfate, appear to have little effect in delaying preterm birth for a day or more. However, the use of maintenance tocolytics, such as oral terbutaline, for women following an episode of preterm labor does not

appear to have benefit in terms of gestational age or infant birthweight. Home monitoring of uterine activity also has no benefit independent of the intervention of nursing care (AHRQ, 2000). As interventions aimed at delaying preterm delivery have not shown conclusive effectiveness, research efforts have moved to the prediction of preterm delivery (ACOG, 2001). For example, the recent use of fetal fibronectin testing to predict the progression of preterm labor to preterm delivery has actually decreased the use of unnecessary interventions (Goepfert et al., 2000). The use of diagnostic technology, then, upholds the principle of utility and decreases the psychosocial stressors of separation from family and community.

The questionable quality of research regarding the efficacy of preterm labor management makes it difficult to draw sound conclusions about effectiveness or risk. To uphold the principle of veracity, researchers must verify evidence with more rigorous studies. Problems with previous studies include small sample size, inconsistent definitions of preterm labor, failure to control for confounding variables, such as maternal medical conditions, and the presence of co-interventions (AHRQ, 2000).

The March of Dimes Prematurity Campaign
On January 30, 2003, the March of Dimes launched a campaign to increase awareness of the growing problem of premature birth. The March of Dimes Prematurity Campaign will invest $75 million over 5 years and will raise new funds to support research into the causes and treatment of prematurity. The campaign will also advocate for an increase of $10 million annually in federally funded research into the causes of prematurity. The goals of the cam-

paign are to increase public awareness of the problem of prematurity from 35 percent to 60 percent and to decrease the rate of preterm birth by at least 15 percent, to no more than 10.1 percent of all births. If the preterm birth rate in 2001 had been 10.1 percent, an estimated 73,000 babies would not have been born prematurely. Table 4 identifies the Prematurity Campaign's five aims.

Many professional groups are partnering with the March of Dimes in this campaign, including AWHONN, ACOG and AAP. In addition, more than 25 professional, consumer and government organizations across the United States have signed on to assist in communicating the campaign's messages to pregnant women, health care professionals and the media. The campaign plans to provide information and education, including continuing education opportunities, to health care providers. These resources are available under *Professionals and Researchers* on the March of Dimes Web site at marchofdimes.com/prematurity.

Table 4. Aims of the March of Dimes Prematurity Campaign

1. Raise public awareness of the problems of prematurity.
2. Educate pregnant women and their families to recognize the signs of preterm labor. Support parents of babies in NICUs.
3. Assist health care practitioners to improve prematurity risk detection and address risk-associated factors.
4. Invest public and private research dollars to identify causes of preterm labor and prematurity and to identify and test promising interventions.
5. Expand access to health insurance to improve prenatal care and infant health outcomes.

Regionalization of Perinatal Care

Regionalization presents ethical dilemmas for providers and pregnant women. Access to perinatal and neonatal technology upholds the idea of social justice. However, geographic isolation and limited health care resources make it difficult for state-of-the-art technology to be available to everyone. In the 1970s, the March of Dimes Committee on Perinatal Health recommended regionalization to increase access to perinatal technology and manage the high costs of technology and staff training (Ryan, 1975). Specific regional centers offering Level III care were designated as high-risk referral centers for complicated pregnancies and ill and preterm newborns. In the 1980s, as regionalization became an established service model, perinatal services began to shift from Level I to Level II care and Level III perinatal centers (Tomich & Anderson, 1990).

Regionalization has contributed to the decreased infant mortality rate in the United States. Intrauterine transfer to a Level III center increases the likelihood that very ill or premature neonates will receive immediate state-of-the-art care (Cordero, Backes & Zuspan, 1982). However, for many pregnant women, transport to a distant Level III medical center is a frightening experience that may settle into weeks or months of separation from family and friends. Unfortunately, assessment of psychosocial impact is not consistently considered part of the care provided to women who are hospitalized for pregnancy complications. Depression screening is rarely conducted, even though the literature shows that women who experience antenatal depression are at increased risk for postpartum depression (Beck, 1996a) and later problems with parenting (Beck, 1996b). At what point is it safe for mothers with complicated pregnan-

Health care decisions made for financial reasons may violate the responsibility to advocate for individual patients.

cies to return from a Level III perinatal center to the care of her community provider? In failing to consistently recognize the psychosocial impact of hospitalization, is actual harm done to the woman? Nonmalfeasance, the obligation to do no harm to patients, is the bottom line for health care providers. Failure to offer holistic plans for perinatal care may, in fact, cause harm.

The principle of utility also must be considered. Over the past two decades, care in perinatal and neonatal services has shifted to higher levels. Much of this is driven by competition between hospitals for market share (Yeast, Poskin, Stockbauer & Shaffer, 1998). Level I hospitals have expanded to provide Level II care, and Level II hospitals are offering Level II+ care. Caution must be taken with financial incentives for maintaining higher patient census, as this could potentially lead to the inappropriate retention of high-risk mothers in Level II facilities. Health care decisions made for financial reasons may violate the responsibility to advocate for individual patients. March of Dimes recommendations for regionalization set criteria for level of care (Ryan, 1975). Level II care should have the ability to stabilize and transfer complicated obstetric cases, including preterm deliveries at <34 weeks gestation. To provide care for premature or ill neonates, a facility should experience more than 2,000 births per year, the volume needed to pay for expensive technology and to maintain skilled staff. Most Level II perinatal care facilities lack this volume. Yeast and colleagues (1998) reported no significant difference in neonatal mortality in Level I vs. Level II centers, and only Level III NICUs demonstrate a trend for improved neonatal mortality rates for very-low-birthweight (VLBW) and extremely-low-birthweight (ELBW) infants.

The trend toward de-regionalization of perinatal services may contribute to adverse outcomes (Phibbs, Bronstein, Buxton & Phibbs, 1996). Long-term financial costs to society may be less if access to perinatal technology is appropriately provided through regionalization. The idea that all providers, all communities and all hospitals can provide high-level perinatal and neonatal technology is simply not feasible from a financial or clinical competency perspective and may actually lead to harm. Strong (2000) argues that in the highly technological era of perinatal health services, low-risk pregnancy care may best be within the scope of practice of certified nurse-midwives, with referral of complicated pregnancies to obstetricians with additional education as maternal/fetal specialists. However, such an approach requires major changes in practice.

In preserving the public trust for the health care professions, the principle of fidelity, the obligation to keep promises, asks that perinatal providers and facilities recognize the limitations of care they provide and make appropriate referrals. Hospital policies regarding appropriate level of care need clear, evidenced-based criteria for referrals.

Maternal/Fetal Conflict Revisited
Maternal/Fetal conflict is a term used by ACOG (1987a) to describe the phenomenon of opposing ethical concerns for the pregnant woman and the fetus. This stance expresses a perceived perinatal dilemma in which the right of the woman to autonomous choice does not appear to be in the best interest of the fetus. Contemporary ethical opinion has moved away from this dichotomous thinking to a relational model in which the fetus cannot be considered separately from the pregnant woman (ACOG, 1987a; Harris, 2000). From a

relational model, it is possible to consider a pregnant woman's well-being and, by association, the well-being of the fetus. However, Hornstra (1998) made clear the dilemma created with maternal/fetal conflict: "There is something unnatural about positing a fetus at odds with its own mother" (p. 10). If providers are to consider the well-being of the fetus, they must first examine the life of the mother in full context. Table 5 identifies questions raised in maternal/fetal conflict.

Substance Abuse in Pregnancy
Prevalence and Consequences
Unhealthy conduct in pregnancy can result in poor perinatal outcomes. Perinatal nurses counsel pregnant women to get early and consistent prenatal care, eat a nutritious diet and refrain from smoking, drinking alcohol or taking drugs or medications not recommended by their health care provider. Most women comply with these recommendations and have healthy pregnancies resulting in healthy term neonates.

However, for some pregnant women, substance use in pregnancy is an overwhelming problem. The ethical concerns raised are complex and numerous. Concerns include the issue of utility in the distribution of available health care resources, maternal autonomy and the provider's obligation to advocate for vulnerable members of society. Annually, approximately 5.5 percent of all neonates are born to mothers who used drugs (including cocaine, marijuana, alcohol or tobacco) during pregnancy (Mathias, 1995).

Table 5. Maternal/Fetal Conflict

- Do the benefits of prolonging a pregnancy to achieve fetal viability justify the risk of complications for the pregnant woman?
- Does the principle of autonomy or self-determination in the presence of completely informed consent override other ethical arguments?
- If the pregnant woman makes a well-informed autonomous choice to decline recommended treatments, do health care providers have further moral responsibility for the fetus?
- Should a woman be compelled to accept treatment for the benefit of the fetus if that benefit presents risk to herself?
- Who decides what is too much maternal risk?
- What constitutes coercion?
- There is limited scientific understanding of why some preterm labor cases resolve with or without treatment, and others proceed to delivery. How can veracity, the responsibility to tell the truth, be upheld if mothers are led to believe that compliance with treatment is the only morally correct choice for the fetus' well-being?
- When appropriate, outpatient or community-based care is more cost-effective, but geographic remoteness from Level III NICU care presents risks for the fetus. At what point is it safe for mothers with complicated pregnancies to return from a Level III perinatal center to the care of the community provider? How is it decided that a pregnant women can be managed as an outpatient vs. an inpatient?
- Are the risks of family disruption and mental health problems for the woman less important than the potential needs of a preterm infant?

A national survey of drug use during pregnancy found that 12.8 percent of women surveyed reported drinking alcohol at some point during their pregnancy (CDC, 2002). Drinking alcohol during pregnancy can cause birth defects, growth problems and fetal alcohol syndrome (FAS), a combination of physical and mental birth defects. In 1999, 12.6 percent of women in the United States smoked during pregnancy (CDC, 2003). Smoking tobacco during pregnancy is a leading cause of low birthweight in the term infant (Aaronson & Macnee, 1989; Lieberman, Gremy, Lang & Cohen, 1994) and is associated with infant mortality, including sudden infant death syndrome (SIDS) (Pollack, Lantz & Frohna, 2000; Schoendorf & Kiely, 1992). The CDC (1995) estimates that $1.4 billion to $2 billion annually can be attributed to the cost of smoking during pregnancy. More than 5 percent of the 4 million women who gave birth in the United States in 1992 used illegal drugs while they were pregnant (Mathias, 1995). Drug use during pregnancy can cause miscarriage, still birth, premature labor, low birthweight and other complications. Babies exposed to drugs in the womb can have addiction problems and withdrawal symptoms and have behavioral, emotional and learning problems later in life.

Substance Use and Ethical Principles
A utilitarian ethical approach questions how providers best care for the most people. The cost to society for health care and education of drug-exposed infants alone is only beginning to be realized. Behnke and colleagues (1997), in a cost analysis of NICU care in Florida, found that when compared (by gestational age, parity, race, maternal age and entry to prenatal care) to non-exposed neonates, cocaine-exposed neonates' health care costs were double. The increased cost was due, in part, to comparably lower birthweights among the cocaine-exposed infants and longer lengths of hospital stay. One factor contributing to longer lengths of stay was the increased social needs of the cocaine-exposed infants and their families. The researchers recommended that addressing social and drug use problems before delivery could decrease costs. To do so, the ethic of caring, with its relational model, must be applied. Antenatal treatment upholds the principle of beneficence for the mother and the fetus.

Maternal substance use during pregnancy seriously affects the well-being of newborns and calls attention to the discussion of fetal rights and society's moral responsibility to its vulnerable members. Unfortunately, the trend has been toward criminalization of prenatal behavior. Attempting to use child abuse and neglect laws, advocates for fetuses and children have supported criminal prosecution of women who abuse substances during pregnancy. The efforts to make charges stick involve controversial interpretation of the law. For example, Jennifer Johnson, a cocaine addict, was found guilty in Florida of delivering drugs to a minor. The minor was her unborn child (*Drug Found in Babies, And Mother is Guilty*, 1989). Another woman, Brenda Vaughan, pled guilty to forging $800 worth of checks and was sentenced to serve out her pregnancy in jail. The prosecutor recommended probation for this first-time offender; however, the judge reasoned that she had screened positive for cocaine in presentencing hearings, and he wanted to protect the fetus (Sachs, 1989). Cases like these continue to stir many ethical questions.

Substance use during pregnancy presents a situation where law and ethics intersect. Advocates of criminal prosecution in prenatal substance use cases have used laws on child abuse as tools for intervention. The Child Abuse Prevention and Treatment Act (42 U.S.C., 1983) requires that states receiving federal grants for developing child abuse treatment and prevention programs must have laws that provide for reporting of known or suspected child abuse and neglect because children of addicted mothers are at risk of neglect and/or abuse (Regan, Ehrlich & Finnegan, 1987). The law in most states requires health care providers to report instances of suspected child abuse or neglect; providers may be held accountable to civil or criminal laws if they do not.

While court-ordered obstetric treatments appear to override maternal autonomy, new legal approaches to influencing maternal behavior have become more common. Based ultimately in the principle of beneficence for the fetus or neonate, courts frequently tie parental rights to the mother's compliance in receiving drug treatment. From the perspective of the ethic of caring and its relational model, women do better in drug rehabilitation if they can keep their children in their care (Hughes et al., 1995).

Maternal behavior allowing injury to the fetus is in direct conflict with the ethical principle of nonmalfeasance, to do no harm. Fear of legal prosecution drives pregnant women with substance abuse problems away from health care providers, where counseling, education, health care surveillance and referral to treatment could improve outcome (upholding the principle of beneficence to the fetus and the pregnant woman). Social health policy in the United States regarding perinatal substance abuse is lacking. Most decisions about how to deal with this health problem are made at the state level. However, addiction is recognized as a primary disease that requires treatment. It will not go away by incarcer-

ating women or by repetitively removing parental rights for each subsequent offspring.

According to the ANA's ethical code, pregnant women who use substances hold claim to the same rights as all other patients, regardless of the nature of the illness (ANA, 2001). The language of conflict is a "social construction" (Chavkin, 1992) and foreign to the natural reality of the maternal/fetal relationship. If women are held accountable for fetal injury related to refusal of medical intervention or substance use during pregnancy, should they also be held accountable for the risk related to secondhand smoke exposure, poor nutritional intake or the decision to stay with abusive partners (Hornstra, 1998)? The application of a relational or care-based ethical model requires that providers understand the decisions of the perinatal patient from the broad perspective of her lived experience. They must invite the perspectives of others in health care and society to avoid personal bias. Ultimately, they must ask what role the patient's sex or race plays in issues of advantage and disadvantage (Harris, 2000).

Research has shown that perinatal nurses generally lack information about substance use during pregnancy. Selleck and Redding (1998) studied 392 perinatal registered nurses in 10 Florida hospitals; they found that the majority had poor understanding of perinatal substance use and that they were likely to hold punitive, judgmental attitudes toward the substance-using mother. From an ethical perspective, nurses have a moral obligation to advocate for the patient. This is difficult to do if the nurse behaves punitively toward the woman. The researchers concluded that the perinatal period presents a unique window of opportunity for intervening in the lives of sub-

Maternal behavior allowing injury to the fetus is in direct conflict with the ethical principle of nonmalfeasance, to do no harm.

stance-using pregnant and postpartum women. It is also important, when considering the ethic of caring, that perinatal nurses view the substance-using pregnant woman from the contextual framework of her life. Application of the ethic of caring assists perinatal nurses in consideration of all forces affecting the pregnant substance user and her ability to change the trajectory of her life.

Traditional treatment approaches historically developed for men who are substance users may not be fully appropriate for women addicts. Woman-centered treatment is an approach that addresses issues not generally part of traditional addiction treatment programs (Reed, 1987). For example, providers must address a woman's responsibilities for childcare and home maintenance and her history of physical and sexual abuse (Woodhouse, 1992). In woman-centered treatment, abstinence is promoted within a safe and empowering environment (Kearney, 1997). Treatment programs for women addicts must include the issues of children and family within a relational model and must address low self-esteem, social isolation and powerlessness. Studies demonstrate that women who are supported in developing and maintaining healthy relationships with their children and other women stay in treatment longer and have better birth outcomes (Finkelstein, 1994; Kearney, 1997). Addiction treatment for women requires a comprehensive approach and the commitment of health care dollars.

Substance addiction is a health care problem and a social problem. The issue of justice must be considered. Is not the most benevolent approach to the fetus of an addicted mother to heal the mother and give the family unit an opportunity to function normally? The challenge for health care providers and all members of society is to do the morally correct thing. Using the criminal justice system to prosecute childbearing addicts does not fully address the issue of beneficence toward the woman. Only a broader social policy addressing treatment needs can do that. Evidence exists that treatment tied to preservation of parental rights and custody increases the likelihood that women will stay in treatment (Hughes et al, 1995).

Court-Ordered Obstetric Treatment
Kolder and colleagues (1987) conducted a national survey of directors of maternal/fetal medicine residency and fellowship programs. Institutions in 26 states and the District of Columbia reported attempts to override maternal refusal of treatment for fetal indications via court order. These cases included court-ordered cesarean sections, hospital detentions and intrauterine transfusions for Rh sensitization. An examination of demographic factors in these cases showed that 81 percent of the pregnant women were women of color, 46 percent were single and 24 percent did not speak English as their primary language. Many were on public assistance. These findings require exploration of how a woman's sociodemographic make-up influences her right to autonomous choice.

The availability of fetal surveillance technology could lead to the assumption that intervention for the welfare of the fetus occurs in the event of fetal distress. However, this assumption is not based in ethical principle. A woman may give permission for fetal surveillance, but not, for example, for an emergency cesarean delivery if the surveillance demonstrates the need. A strong ethical obligation exists in health care to respect the autonomous choice of the patient. This is the concept behind informed consent. However, in perinatal health care, this position is not clear cut. The confounding factor is consideration for the fetus. Does a pregnant woman's refusal of medical treatment that would benefit the fetus constitute a violation of the principle of beneficence? Some argue that a pregnant woman's decision to maintain a pregnancy commits her ethically to the preservation of fetal well-being. In fact, most pregnant women do what they can to preserve fetal well-being by following recommended medical treatments and living a lifestyle that is conducive to fetal growth and development. However, for some women, pregnancy is not a welcomed event, and maternal social conditions do not provide a nurturing environment for pregnancy. In these cases, the result is a less-than-healthy or at-risk pregnancy. When a pregnancy is at risk, the judicial system may decide to override a pregnant woman's right to autonomous choice to protect the fetus.

The Roe v. Wade decision added fuel to the argument for forced treatments by identifying the legal responsibility to the viable fetus. Moderate ethicists sought a balance of maternal and fetal rights (Chervenak & McCullough, 1985; Strong, 1991). Arguments about court-ordered treatment of pregnant women for fetal indications center on the ethical principles of autonomy for the mother, veracity about the limited ability to predict individual long-term outcomes and beneficence toward the fetus. One position is that court-ordered interventions are never justified if they violate the woman's right to self-determination (King, 1991; Ryan, 1990). Another position is that a court-ordered intervention is justified in rare, exceptional circumstances when it "poses insignificant health risks to the woman or would promote the interests in life and health, and [if] there are compelling reasons to over-ride her autonomy" (Strong, 1991, p. 861). This view conflicts with ACOG's position that there is almost never a reason to coerce or force a pregnant woman to undergo any treatment or intervention against her will. To do so limits maternal freedom of choice, threatens the doctor-patient relationship and violates the principles underlying informed consent (ACOG, 1987b).

The incidence of court-ordered interventions for medical treatment has decreased. Court orders do little for the welfare of the pregnant woman or her fetus. An example is the case of 26-year-old Angela Carder (Macklin, 1995). Ms. Carder had metastatic cancer and wanted to maintain her pregnancy. As her health deteriorated, she entered George Washington University Hospital in Washington, DC for supportive care. Physicians determined that Ms. Carder had little time left and that the fetal condition had deteriorated, and they proposed a cesarean delivery. However, Ms. Carder was ambivalent. The hospital, against the wishes of physicians and the family, sought a court order to determine treatment. The fetus was appointed legal representation, and the court ordered the surgery. The fetus died 2½ hours after surgery. Ms. Carder died two days later.

Court orders do little for the welfare of the pregnant woman or her fetus.

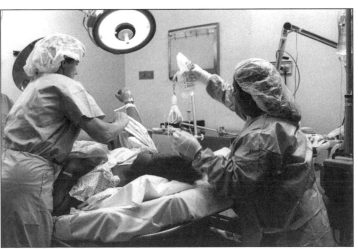

Maternal-fetal conflict is a misnomer; it is, in fact, more a question of maternal-physician conflict.

Reaction from the Carder case has enforced the rights of pregnant women. A Washington, DC appeals court vacated the decision regarding Ms. Carder, meaning that the decision could not be used as a legal precedent for future cases (Macklin, 1995). Law is the only means, in most societies, that can regulate the moral code of social behavior. The Court of Appeals decision in this case is an example of using the law to enforce ethical principle (Laganá, 2000). Additionally, the hospital adopted a policy that places the autonomy of pregnant women before other ethical considerations (Macklin, 1995).

Maternal-fetal conflict is a misnomer; it is, in fact, more a question of maternal-physician conflict (King, 1991; Ryan, 1990). A physician may view a pregnant woman's decision to forego medical treatment that may improve fetal outcome as irrational, thereby increasing the physician's moral obligation to protect the fetus (King, 1991). Calling a competent adult's decision irrational does not morally justify the overriding of that individual's right to self-determination. Additionally, the right to refuse medical treatment is recognized in the U.S. Constitution's *Bill of Rights* under the right to privacy (Antoine, 1989).

The idea that a parent should submit to the risk of therapy for the welfare of the fetus, such as the risk of major surgery in a cesarean section, finds no parallel in parental responsibility. For example, there is no legal precedent for demanding a parent donate a kidney to a child in renal failure. The acknowledged uncertainty of fetal diagnosis and outcome raises ethical concern about legal attempts to override a pregnant woman's right to autonomy. An example is the 1981 case in Georgia of Jefferson v. Griffin Spalding City Hospital. Jessie Mae Jefferson was diagnosed with a complete placenta previa and refused to consent to a planned cesarean section birth at the onset of labor, stating that her religious faith would heal her body. A court awarded temporary custody of her unborn child to the State of Georgia and ordered her to obtain an ultrasound exam with a subsequent cesarean section if the placenta previa persisted. The court based its decision on the testimony of the attending physician who gave the fetus <1 percent chance of surviving a vaginal birth. The court ruled that the unborn child merited protection under the law as a minor and found that the state's duty to protect the unborn fetus outweighed the violation of Jefferson's bodily integrity. The motion was denied, citing Roe v. Wade and other cases as support for the decision. Jessie Mae Jefferson refused to comply and experienced an uneventful vaginal delivery of a normal healthy infant (Annas, 1982).

The threat of court-ordered treatment of pregnant women for fetal indications raises many concerns. When a woman fears her health care provider, or when she does not perceive health care services as beneficent, she may avoid health care altogether. Is rare, poor fetal outcome worth the price for denying the rights of competent adults to self-determination, regardless of medical condition, ethnic background or socioeconomic status? Providers can obtain informed consent only in a supportive environment where patients can hear and process information (Childress, 1990). Many women refuse recommended treatment out of fear or misunderstanding. If providers believe that all competent adults have a right to informed choice, then they must create an environment in which pregnant women can make choices that uphold not only their right to autonomy, but also the principle of beneficence toward the fetus. Provision One of the ANA's (2001) *Code of Ethics for Nurses with Interpretive Statements* states, "The nurse, in all professional relationships, practices with compassion and respect for the inherent dignity, work and uniqueness of every individual, unrestricted by considerations of social or economic status, personal attributes or the nature of health problems" (p. 7).

Reproductive Technology and Genetics

Improved understanding of the causes of human infertility, coupled with the unfolding of the human genome in the late 20th century, has led to a surge of new reproductive technology. With that technology comes the promise of doing profound good, such as the elimination of genetically linked diseases. However, new technology raises new ethical questions—where, if anywhere, should lines of constraint be drawn? Increased genetic understanding influences reproductive technology. As the two areas meet, the possibilities for manipulation of human offspring become more challenging from an ethical perspective. Ethical arguments include equality in access to and application of genetic knowledge and reproductive technology, utility in the high cost of reproductive technology, the importance of confidentiality and the right to refuse genetic testing or to act on its findings.

Infertility and Assisted Reproductive Technology. The CDC's 1995 *National Family Survey* (CDC, 1997) determined that 2 percent of 60 million women of childbearing age surveyed consulted with a health care provider for an infertility-related problem, and 13 percent had some lifetime experience with infertility medical services ranging from counseling to assisted reproductive technology (ART). The

CDC defines ART as all fertility treatments involving the handling of both human egg and sperm; the CDC'S definition does not include artificial insemination, in which only sperm is manipulated, or drug-stimulated egg production, which involves only the ovum (CDC, 2000a). ART does include in vitro fertilization (IVF), gamete intrafallopian transfer (GIFT) and zygote intrafallopian transfer (ZIFT). These involve laboratory collection of ovum and sperm and reintroduction in various stages of fertilization into a female reproductive tract. GIFT and ZIFT both require laproscopy. The world was introduced in 1978 to IVF with the birth of Baby Louise Brown, the first test tube baby (Francis & Nosck, 1988). Her life gave hope to millions of infertile women and their partners and created a consumer demand for ART that appears to be limited only by financial barriers and the consumer's desire to become pregnant.

Like sperm, eggs can be donor or non-donor. Implanted embryos may be donor or non-donor, fresh or frozen. As ART has advanced, success rates have increased in the manipulation of the ovum (oocyte) and sperm. For example, intra-cytoplasmic sperm injection (ICSI) is used in some cases

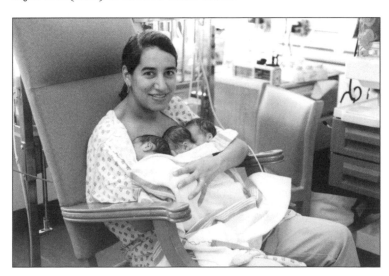

for abnormal or low sperm counts to actually puncture the zona pelucida surface of the ovum and inject the sperm. While ICSI for male fertility appears to slightly increase the chance of fertilization of the ovum, it does not appear to increase the number of live births (CDC, 2000a). Transfer of thawed embryos appears to result in fewer live births (19.3 percent) than with fresh embryos (30.8 percent), but it is less expensive and less invasive because the egg retrieval portion of the cycle is not needed. In 1998, 90.4 percent of ART cycles used non-donor eggs or embryos; of these, 13 percent used non-donor frozen embryos (CDC, 2000a).

A 1992 federal law requires the CDC to annually report ART cycle success rates. The CDC expects all ART clinics and providers to report success rates. The ART cycle includes egg retrieval, laboratory manipulation of the egg and sperm, transfer of the embryo to a uterus, pregnancy and live birth. The 2000 CDC report indicates that of the 62,000 cycles started in 1998 with fresh non-donor eggs or embryos, 15,000 (approximately 25 percent) resulted in live births. Of the clinical pregnancies that occurred (30.5 percent of the cycles), roughly half resulted in single-ton births, and less than one-third resulted in multiple-infant births. The remainder resulted in spontaneous or therapeutic pregnancy termination or stillbirth (CDC, 2000a). When birth of a live infant is not attainable using non-donor eggs or embryos, donor eggs and embryos are an option. Delayed childbearing often necessitates the use of donor eggs. Maternal age is the most important factor associated with ART success with non-donor eggs or embryos—both pregnancy rates and live births rapidly decline after the age of 35 (CDC, 2000a).

All forms of ART present ethical questions regarding cost, efficacy, benefits and risks for infertile women or couples, donors, surrogates and potential offspring. Ethical issues become more evident with the use of donor eggs or embryos. Approximately 10 percent of ART cycles in 1998 involved the use of donor eggs. Most women in these cases were 37 years old or older. ART is more successful with donor eggs than with fresh, non-donor eggs; women of all ages who use donor eggs experience live birth rates comparable with (or higher than) rates of women in their mid-30s or younger who use their own eggs (CDC, 2000a). With egg donation, donors can undergo an egg-retrieval procedure and, in return, receive reimbursement that is normally capped at $5,000 per procedure, an amount that might be seen as coercive considering the youth and relatively lower income levels of donors (Larkin, 2000). Donor advocacy usually consists of informed consent before relinquishing all parental rights to offspring via contractual agreement; clinics vary in informed consent policies. The American Society for Reproductive Medicine (ASRM) (2000a) recommends counseling for the donor that includes information on physical and psychological risks and the need for medical follow-up. Usually, a woman or a couple can review anonymous profiles of donors, including information on height, weight, eye and hair color and athletic and academic ability, to make a decision about the use of donor eggs.

ART also raises ethical concerns because of the growing technological capability to manipulate genetic material. The use of donor sperm or eggs that provides a pregnancy for a couple appears to uphold the principle of beneficence. However, issues may arise related to lack of a genetic link between the resulting infant and the father in the case of sperm donation; in the case of a donor egg, there is no genetic link with the mother. Initially, the use of donor eggs or sperm was the basis of ART. The ability now exists for transfer of maternal genetic material into younger donor eggs, thus providing a genetic link with the infertile woman. This transfer of genetic material is the basis of reproductive cloning. Additionally, utilizing available technology to procreate is a personal choice that is supported by the principle of autonomy. If the infertile couple is able to become pregnant, carry the pregnancy to term and fulfill the desire to become parents, the principle of beneficence is upheld. A similar argument can be made for all infertility treatments.

A case involving ART to provide a pregnancy for a 63-year-old woman (NOVA, 2001) raised concerns about risk to the subsequent offspring. Arceli Keh wanted to have a baby, but she was menopausal. Keh represented herself to her reproductive specialist as a 50-year-old, meeting the maximum age limit for ART. After hormonal therapy to ready her uterus for implantation, the fifth IVF cycle, using a donor egg and her husband's sperm, led to the live birth of a normal baby girl. The ethical concern was one of nonmalfeasance for the child. With parents the age of most grandparents, critics asked how long will the parents live to care for the child? Humans are living longer every year, so the likelihood of the Kehs living until their daughter's adulthood is a real possibility. But, to avoid an unwarranted burden on society and injury to the child, should regulations require older ART recipients to designate replacement parents in the event of their demise? Most clinics self-police this situation by denying ART to older individuals. Advocates for reproductive rights, as well as society in general, may not yet be ready for this level of encroachment on individual autonomy.

The principle of justice is violated when the right to life is not universal for all. ART must also be considered from the principles of justice and utility due to its exorbitant cost. Because of the expense, ART is not available to all members of society. However, not all infertility treatments require the technological sophistication and expense of ART. Less than 5 percent of women seeking assistance for infertility eventually use ART; most women who become pregnant following access to infertility services do so without ART (Association of Women's Health, Obstetric and Neonatal Nursing [AWHONN], 2000). Large disparities exist in health insurance coverage for infertility treatment. While many states have laws requiring insurance companies to cover some form of infertility treatment, benefits are inconsistent (CDC, 1999a). Treatment available only to the privileged violates the principle of justice. Additionally, the principle of utility (bringing the greatest good or happiness to the greatest number of people) is not upheld in a therapy that is too costly for most people. Where might social resources be more equitably spent? Adoption, once the primary route to parenthood for infertile couples, has taken a secondary place to ART. As a society, what does this say about our willingness to care for vulnerable and parentless children with unknown intrauterine environments or genetic codes?

As with all new technologies, the outcome of ART is not fully known. The truth is that ART is limited in its success in producing healthy births (CDC, 2000a). Women and their partners need to see the figures and make informed choices about pursuing this technology. White (1992) noted that, from an ethical perspective, perhaps the most important role for nurses working in the area of reproductive medicine is that of advocacy concern-

If the infertile couple is able to become pregnant, carry the pregnancy to term and fulfill the desire to become parents, the principle of beneficence is upheld.

ing informed consent. The moral challenge is to accomplish this advocacy in a clinical arena that is increasingly market-driven. Thousands of women have been assisted in their efforts to procreate through reproductive technology. This benefit cannot be underestimated. However, complex issues surrounding this technology are changing the moral fabric of society and must be diligently analyzed.

Surrogacy. The surrogate mother is a woman who, through artificial insemination or IVF, is impregnated for the purpose of carrying an infant to term for another woman. This is an especially benevolent approach for women who, for medical reasons such as Rokitansky Syndrome (normal gonads, but agenesis of the uterus and vagina), are unable to carry a pregnancy (Beski, Gorgy, Venka, Craft & Edmonds, 2000). The ovum can be from the surrogate, a donor or the woman who will legally parent the infant. The surrogate mother can be a friend or relative of the legal parents or an unknown individual recruited into a surrogacy contract.

Autonomy in reproductive rights for both the surrogate and the contracting couple is upheld. However, beyond the argument of individual rights is a concern for the offspring in surrogacy contracts. For example, Baby M was a female born in 1985 as a result of a surrogacy contract. William Stern, Baby M's biological father, and his wife contracted with Mary Beth Whitehead to carry a pregnancy conceived of his artificially inseminated sperm and the surrogate mother's ovum. The surrogacy contract stipulated that the Sterns would adopt the offspring at birth and pay hospital expenses and a $10,000 surrogacy fee. After delivery, Whitehead refused to relinquish the infant. The court system was called in to decide who should keep Baby M (Cahill, 1988).

With the help of surrogates, infertile couples can, in most cases, have a baby with a biological connection to one or more parents. This upholds the principle of beneficence. The surrogate mother has the right to enter into a surrogacy contract, upholding the principle of autonomy. However, the Baby M case highlighted the moral dilemma created when a woman attempts to relinquish her autonomy as a parent. The surrogacy contract spelled out Whitehead's agreement to be artificially inseminated with Stern's sperm, see designated obstetricians, abstain from lifestyle activities that might threaten the pregnancy or fetal development and, at birth, release any claim to parenthood. But, ultimately, the court had to decide the power of a written contract to override the principle of autonomy. The final decision recognized parental rights for both Stern and Whitehead but awarded custody of Baby M to the biological father, with visitation rights for the biological mother.

The court decision also addressed moral responsibility to the non-autonomous members of society, in this case, Baby M. In the judgment of the court, the welfare of Baby M could be best served in the home and custody of the biological father. The degree to which the biological father's superior financial stability contributed to the court's decision was unclear and raised the question of justice to the less financially stable biologic mother. In addition, the court addressed the principle of nonmalfeasance by considering which custody arrangement would best protect the psychological welfare of Baby M. By providing visitation to the surrogate mother, the court ensured that, in part, the reality of Baby M's parenthood would be known. But should a child grow up knowing the details of his or her conception? How does a legally constructed, split family affect a child's welfare?

Taken to the other extreme is the case of Luanne and John Buzzanca (Annas, 1998). The Buzzancas contracted with a surrogate mother to gestate an embryo using donor eggs and donor sperm. However, before the birth of baby girl Jaycee, the Buzzancas separated. John Buzzanca rejected parental responsibility. The surrogate mother argued that she never intended to parent the child. As there was no genetic link with any of the involved parties, a court case ensued to determine parental responsibility for the newborn. The judge found that the newborn was legally parentless. The idea of a parentless child is morally untenable. An appeals court reversed the decision. According to California law, a father must consent to the artificial insemination of his wife and is legally the parent; the surrogate contract held the Buzzancas to the same spirit of the law. Parental responsibility was assigned to Luanne and John Buzzanca (Buzzanca v. Buzzanca, 1998).

In the Buzzanca case, the judge made a strong appeal for regulatory law in the area of surrogacy. Others hold that the decision to become a surrogate is protected by the principle of autonomy and associated reproductive rights. Van Zyl and Van Kiekark (2000), in a qualitative study of the meaning of surrogate motherhood, found that women enter into surrogacy contracts for diverse reasons. They argued that efforts to seriously restrict or ban surrogacy contracts violates a woman's right to enter into contractual agreements and imposes culturally and socially constructed views of motherhood.

Stored, unused, frozen embryos raise other ethical questions. Many clinics ask clients to designate long-term plans for created embryos. Embryos designated for disposal if not used for implantation raise a special concern.

Embryo freezing and its associated moral and ethical dilemma was made clear in 1981 when an Australian couple was killed in a plane crash (Press, 1984). Part of the couple's legacy was frozen embryos. Legal debate over the rights of the embryos to inheritance ensued—what happens when technology makes it possible for children to be born after the death of their biological parents?

In another case, Maureen and Steven Kass experienced five egg retrievals and nine IVF embryo transfers. None were successful. Maureen's sister agreed to serve as surrogate, and extensive informed consents were signed, including consent for disposal of unused, stored, frozen embryos for appropriate research. No surrogate pregnancy occurred, and the couple divorced. Maureen successfully sued for custody of the remaining frozen embryos for future implantation (Kass v. Kass, 1997). On appeal, the courts overturned the decision on the grounds that the contract for disposal was binding (Annas, 1998).

Multiple Gestation and Fetal Reduction. ART often results in multiple births. Use of ovulation-stimulating drugs and implantation of multiple embryos increase the incidence of multiple pregnancies. Multiple pregnancies are at increased risk of preterm labor and preterm delivery. Multiples are three to five times more likely to be admitted to the NICU, and multiple births are more costly because of longer hospital stays for mothers and infants (Bowers, 1998). The CDC (2000a) reported that, in 1998, 11 percent of ART pregnancies using fresh, non-donor eggs or embryos were triplets or more, and 28 percent were twins. Forty-seven percent of the cycles involved the transfer of four or more embryos (CDC, 2000a).

The United States is one of the few Western countries without established social policy to comprehensively support women during pregnancy and after delivery.

A few high-profile cases have caught national media attention. In 1985, Ms. Frustaci delivered septuplets following the use of medication to increase ovulation. Of the seven infants, three survived with prematurity-related morbidity. The Frustacis sued the fertility clinic for not monitoring the number of ovum folicles before artificial insemination and were awarded $2.7 million (*Promise of Seven Babies*, 1997). In 1997, following the use of the fertility drug Metrodin, Ms. McCaughey delivered septuplets (*Four Boys, Three Girls*, 1997). This case raised questions about the morality of creating a pregnancy so at-risk that the seven preterm infants and their mother required extensive and expensive medical care (Klotzko, 1998).

Fetal reduction decreases the number of fetuses and the risks associated with multiples (Berkowitz et al., 1988). Fetal reduction is used to selectively abort one or more fetuses to provide for a twin gestation. Studies show improved outcome when quadruplet gestations are reduced to twin gestations. Reductions from triplet to twin gestations are more controversial, as outcomes are not markedly different from non-reduced triplets (Melgar, Rosenfield, Rawlinson & Greenberg, 1991; Porrelo, Burke & Hendrix, 1991). Criticism of fetal reduction has led to decreasing the number of implanted embryos. Fetal reduction upholds the principle of beneficence by promoting longer gestation in surviving fetuses and by decreasing maternal complications associated with preterm labor. However, the "reduced" fetus (or fetuses) cannot share in this benefit. How is it decided which fetus will die? Does the sex of the fetus come into the decision-making process? It is unethical to eliminate a fetus based solely on sex.

Since Roe v. Wade, societal attitude toward reproductive rights has led to abortion debates in the U.S. legislature and courts. Attitudes have polarized into two camps—the right to life and the right to choice. While the moral dilemma of abortion is hotly debated, women who forego abortion and assume the financial and emotional responsibilities of unexpected or multiple pregnancies receive little financial or social support. The United States is one of the few Western countries without established social policy to comprehensively support women during pregnancy and after delivery (Stotland, 1990).

Preimplantation Genetic Diagnosis. The Human Genome Project (HGP) began in 1990 following years of international efforts, supported by the March of Dimes, to map the human genome. In the United States, HGP research is sponsored by the National Human Genome Research Institute at the National Institutes of Health, in conjunction with the Office of Biological and Environmental Research at the Department of Energy. HGP findings indicate that at the DNA level, humans are 99.9 percent similar. The human genome contains an estimated 40,000 protein-coding genes. The complexity of human genes raises questions about diseases with multi-gene links (Carrico, 2001). Genetics research has historically focused on the role of gene mutation on human disease and the role of genes in turning on or off proteins that influence health. For example, scientists at the Salk Institute in San Francisco are studying the roles of a set of master genes that are critical for embryonic limb formation (March of Dimes, 2000). Once a protein is expressed, environmental factors influence that expression. The Human Genome Project fuels further work on basic genetics questions and will hopefully present approaches for treating genetically determined human diseases.

Preimplantation genetic diagnosis (PGD) is a technique that allows for analysis of embryos before implantation. Entire cells can be removed from a developing embryo and analyzed without killing the developing embryo. The healthiest embryos can be selected for implantation, increasing the likelihood of success. PGD aimed at the avoidance of sex-linked genetic disorders upholds the principle of beneficence by preventing a life of suffering. However, PGD gender selection related to the desire for a male or female offspring raises the question of gender discrimination. Even the concept of family balancing (a desire for male and female offspring) upholds both beneficence and parental autonomy (American Society for Reproductive Medicine [ASRM], 2001). However, once an embryo exists, deposition of unwanted embryos raises ethical concerns. While different ethical arguments exist concerning the rights of the fetus, some argue that the embryo is human life and has the moral right to protection. No laws exist that uphold human rights of the unimplanted embryo. Legal precedent treats embryos as property. Parents currently can dispose of unused embryos as desired. Many divorce proceedings have dealt with decisions about what to do with frozen embryos.

Preconception gender selection is a technique that neatly avoids arguments concerning embryos. Preconception gender selection involves microsort techniques that detect minute size differences in sperm related to the X chromosome, with an accurate prediction rate of 90 percent for females and 70 percent for males (NOVA, 2001). Is it immoral for parents to choose the gender of their children? In many cultures, a male child is preferred. In the United States, this is not a current social trend. Gender preference for

male children in China, coupled with restrictive social health policies allowing for only one offspring, has created an orphanage system filled with unwanted girls. A social health policy aimed at curbing China's skyrocketing population growth was a utilitarian effort to plan for adequate resources. Parental autonomy, coupled with the social policy, produced many female orphans.

The principle of social justice is based on equal rights to all members of society. PGD, with all of its possibilities for improving the genetic quality of human beings, is among the greatest threats to social justice. The genetic heterogeneity that exists among human beings is a social equalizer, providing the opportunity to escape a less-than-optimal environment. Taken to a reasonable extreme, PGD could lead to offspring free of illness or selected for certain desirable personal characteristics. Such genetic engineering could provide social advantage for some, as those without access to genetic screening or genetic engineering would not be able to compete with genetically engineered individuals. Dr. Lee Silver, a molecular biologist at Princeton University, has concerns about genetic engineering, which could eventually create such genetic class differences that mating could become a problem. In essence, genetic engineering could lead to multiple human species (NOVA, 2001).

The ASRM (1999) identified concerns regarding PGD, including sex selection, as "the potential for inherent gender discrimination, inappropriate control over nonessential characteristics of children, unnecessary medical burdens and costs for parents and inappropriate and potentially unfair use of limited medical resources" (p.596). However, the same authors argued

No laws exist that uphold human rights of the unimplanted embryo. Legal precedent treats embryos as property.

that, in a society where gender equality exists, gender selection in reproductive medicine would not pose the threat of gender discrimination. Instead, reproductive choice might be based on an equal valuing of female and male children and the desire to rear children of each sex (ASRM, 2001).

Cloning. The first publicized, cloned mammal was Dolly, a sheep cloned by Scottish scientists in 1997. The procedure involved the removal of the nucleus from a mammary gland cell of an adult ewe. The mammary gland cell, a differentiated cell (unlike a stem cell), contained a complete genetic code and could be manipulated in the laboratory to full genetic expression. The nucleus was introduced into the enucleated ovum of another sheep, and the newly reconstructed cell received a growth-stimulating electrical charge. The resulting embryo implanted into the uterus of another sheep developed into Dolly, an identical genetic copy of the donor ewe. While remarkable, the procedure's effectiveness was shadowed by the 276 failures preceding Dolly's birth (Greenlee, 2000). Improvement in the procedure has since resulted in the successful cloning of other species.

A clone can consist of a single cell or an entire organism. Two procedures can make a clone: somatic cell nuclear transfer (SCNT) and blastomere splitting. Blastomere splitting resulting in identical twins is an example of spontaneously occurring human clones. Scientists have accomplished artificial blastomere splitting.

There are three types of cloning: embryonic cloning, therapeutic cloning and reproductive cloning. All three raise different ethical concerns. Embryonic cloning involves the enucleation of blastomeres and transfer of those nuclei into same-species oocytes. The resulting multiple identical embryos

are implanted into the uteri of the animal model to create identical individuals for research. This type of cloning is considered unethical for use in humans because it blatantly violates the principle of human self-determination and illustrates a worst-case scenario for arguments against cloning. Embryonic cloning has been used in non-human primates and other animals (Soules, 2001).

Therapeutic cloning is the technology used for development of embryos for stem cells. Embryonic stem cells are genetically identical to the donor and can be used for differentiation into replacement tissue (Soules, 2001). While highly controversial, therapeutic cloning has the potential for organ and tissue transplantation and eliminates the risk of antigenic rejection.

SCNT, as used to create Dolly, is reproductive cloning. The purpose of SCNT is to create a pregnancy. SCNT, still an experimental procedure, provides the possibility of securing a genetic link for infertile couples with a technology that challenges ethical norms by the very nature of its possibilities. Unlike the natural blending of two genetic lineages, SCNT is an asexual procedure that does not require the genetic material of two individuals. The ASRM (2000b) calls it a "dramatic departure from natural or assisted conception" (p. 874) in that it is, more accurately, replication rather than reproduction.

In 1997, the National Bioethics Advisory Board found that human cloning is unethical, and President Clinton issued an executive order barring the use of federal funds for research on human cloning (ANA 2000). However, demand for cloning technology from those who want to recover lost loved ones is creating underground funding in the private sector (Alexander, 2001).

Cloning is perched on the proverbial slippery slope of ethical dilemma. While many arguments offer benevolent solutions to human problems of infertility, loss or illness, others point to the potential for abuse of new reproductive technologies. The National Advisory Board on Ethics in Reproduction (1994) cited reasons for cloning that ranged from improved chances of initiating pregnancy in IVF treatment to retaining an identical twin embryo for the purpose of future gestation and organ or tissue transplants to its living twin. Ethical arguments in favor of human cloning include the right to reproductive freedom, the right to free scientific inquiry and patient demand (Soules, 2001). Cloning upholds the principle of beneficence by allowing avoidance of genetically linked illness or providing pregnancy for infertile couples who bear genetic relatedness (ASRM, 2000b).

While concerns about the safety of SCNT for human cloning make it unethical under the principle of non-malfeasance, ethical arguments against human cloning are based in autonomy and the risk to human individuality and uniqueness (Hopkins, 1998). Reproductive cloning has not been proven safe in animal models. Cardiopulmonary and placentation problems and pregnancy losses are common (Soules, 2001). Risks for physical and psychological well-being of the cloned individual are unknown. There is no way of predicting if a human clone will be normal. Ultimately, the risk exists that selective cloning will result in preferential treatment of individual qualities, which could lead to discrimination against members of society based on the very uniqueness and individuality that is currently protected by moral norms. For example, physical attributes, such as hair color or personality traits, could become a symbol of superiority. Another concern regarding cloning is the possibility of commercial development of clones for the purpose of stem cell harvesting.

While research atrocities, such as the Tuskegee syphilis experiment, changed societal beliefs about the rights of individuals to informed and voluntary consent (National Commission for the Protection of Human Subjects of Biomedical and Behavioral Research, 1979), the flood of new knowledge and technological advancement demands that society give serious thought to technological research. The undetermined trajectory of genetic and reproductive technology calls for the increased vigilance of a moral society. What was once considered science fiction is now science fact. Reproductive medicine clinics are already using techniques similar to SCNT.

Cloning research has limited federal oversight, largely because laws prohibit its federal funding. However, research continues at an accelerated rate in the private sector. Without public oversight, it is difficult for a society to control cloning technology. The ANA's position paper on human cloning (2000) cited the International Council of Nurses position that "human cloning violates the right to one's unique genetic identity and dignity" and supported a vigorous national and international debate on cloning.

Stem Cell Research. Scientists first isolated human stem cells from embryos discarded by reproductive clinics and from fetal cadavers (Meslin, 2000). Stem cells can differentiate into other tissues and offer great promise for regeneration of damaged or aging human tissue. Stem cells are found in embryonic, as well as adult, human tissue (National Institutes of Health, 2001). They have also been isolated in umbilical cords (March of Dimes, 2002b).

Ethical arguments in favor of human cloning include the right to reproductive freedom, the right to free scientific inquiry and patient demand.

Neonatal technology raises ethical questions about quality of life and distribution of neonatal resources.

A recent development is the commercial banking of cord blood, which indicates the therapeutic, as well as economic, value of stem cells. While the use of cord blood for stem cells is experimental, commercial ventures are marketing cord blood banking to new parents for future use by the infant, family members or other non-related individuals. Cost and storage limitations are issues that providers should discuss with parents during the informed consent process (Pinch, 2001).

Questions exist regarding informed consent in the use of stored, biological samples for genetics research (Clayton et al, 1995). Many believe that increasing knowledge is generally good for individuals and society. However, using stored, biological samples that were collected for individual diagnostic work-up may violate the patient's right to informed consent. Federal regulations regarding the use of stored biological specimens exempt requirements for the protection of human subjects if identifiers are irretrievably removed from the samples and if the specimens were collected before the start of the research (Clayton et al, 1995).

The use of fetal tissue from aborted fetuses designated for stem cell research creates another ethical dilemma that goes beyond the argument of right to life for the fetus. The question becomes one of wrongful life, when pregnancies are conceived and aborted for the purpose of producing stem cells. In August 2001, President Bush agreed to allow federal funding for stem cell research on aborted fetuses and stored embryos but restricted funding for the development of embryos to serve as sources for stem cells.

Informed consent from donors to use embryos or fetal tissue in research may be inadequate by itself to protect human rights. Privacy and confiden-

tiality must be considered. Legislation is needed to protect children who are created with new technology. It may be necessary to impose regulations and legal oversight in development and application of reproductive technology. The National Bioethics Advisory Commission argued for a unified, comprehensive federal policy to provide research oversight (National Bioethics Advisory Commission, 2001). French philosopher, scientist and Jesuit priest Pierre Teilhard de Chardin (1881-1955) wrote prophetically about the need to consider the dilemmas faced as a society:

"Yet though we may exalt research and derive enormous benefit from it, with what pettiness of spirit, poverty of means and general haphazardness do we pursue the truth in the world today? Have we ever given serious thought to the predicament we are in? The truth is that, as children of a transitional period, we are neither fully conscious of, nor in full control of, the new powers that have been unleashed" (Teilhard de Chardin, 1976, p. 278-279).

Neonatal Technology and Research

The emergence of neonatal technologies has dramatically improved the survival of extremely low birthweight infants. Neonatal technology raises ethical questions about quality of life and distribution of neonatal resources.

Evaluating Outcomes

New neonatal techniques have contributed to improvements in morbidity and mortality rates among term and preterm infants, and experimental therapies have contributed to the decrease in mortality in ELBW infants. However, these developments have heightened concerns about the limits of viability. Survival of infants born at 23 weeks gestation is approximately 20 percent, while infants born at 28 weeks have survival rates that exceed 90 percent (Muraskas et al, 1999). Long-term outcomes for ELBW infants are ambiguous and uncertain. Providers must consider ethical implications of failed interventions in ELBW infants and moral consequences of further treatment.

Some medical centers encourage discontinuation of life support for ELBW infants who, despite initial therapies, fail to have adequate oxygenation in the early hours following birth. Parents' wishes for initial resuscitation of an ELBW infant should be respected, particularly for infants who weigh <600 g with a gestational age of 23 to 24 weeks. However, problems associated with the treatment of ELBW infants raise questions about interventions that might be medically futile (Muraskas et al., 1999). From a utilitarian standpoint, intervention withdrawal is justifiable from a perspective of medical futility and from the inability to uphold the principle of beneficence.

The Neonatal Donor

Laura Campo did not have medical insurance and did not seek prenatal care until the 24th week of pregnancy. She learned when she was 8 months pregnant that her baby was anencephalic. Because the diagnosis was made so late in pregnancy, she could not have an abortion. Ms. Campo heard about anencephalic infant organ donation on a talk show. She decided to bring the fetus to term to donate the organs. Because an anencephalic infant often has a swollen head, vaginal delivery risks fetal demise and damage to organs for transplantation. Ms. Campo understood that she would need a cesarean delivery. Baby Theresa was born on March 21, 1992 in Fort Lauderdale, Florida.

Providers expected Baby Theresa to die within minutes after birth, but she did not. Baby Theresa had to be declared brain dead before her organs could be donated. Her parents asked that she be declared brain dead. However, Baby Theresa did not meet the criteria for brain death under Florida law, and the neonatologist refused to remove the organs (Pence, 2000). Pictures of Baby Theresa showing a beautiful baby girl wearing a pink knitted cap that covered the top half of her head were distributed to the press. Underneath the cap were no skin, no skull and no cerebrum.

The parents appealed to the Florida circuit court to rule that Baby Theresa was dead. The judge ruled that she was unable to authorize taking Baby Theresa's life to save another. The couple appealed to the Florida District Court of Appeals, which affirmed the circuit court's decision. As the case grew in publicity, the parents appealed to the Florida Supreme Court. The Florida Supreme Court lacked constitutional authority to hear the case because the District Court of Appeals had ruled that it was not of "great public importance" (Pence, 2000).

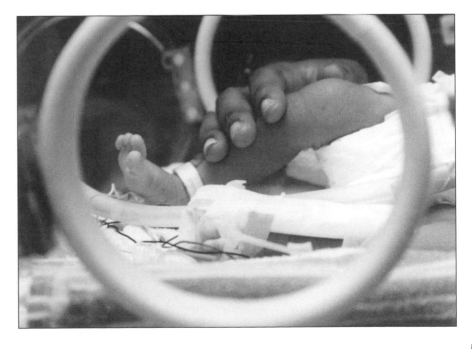

On March 29, Baby Theresa's organs began to fail. By the time the respirator was removed, the organs were unusable for transplantation. Baby Theresa died on March 30, and her organs were useless for transplantation. The case of Baby Theresa raises questions about the criteria used for infants as donors.

With the increasing need for organ procurement in this country, the value and worth of the anencephalic infant has become a moral dilemma. Procuring organs from a brain dead infant does not present the same ethically challenging issue as procuring organs from an anencephalic infant. Anencephalic infants have a functioning brainstem at birth and some reflex activity that remains viable for a short period of time. Without medical intervention, the anencephalic infant is not able to perfuse the body's organs and, therefore, expires. To maintain the perfusion of the anencephalic infant on life support to protect organs for procurement creates an ethical dilemma. The criteria for brain death under a week of age are not firm, making prolonged life support for these infants controversial (Loewy, 1996).

At the center of the controversy is the value or primary worth of anencephalics. Without the neocortex, the anencephalic infant lacks the capacity for higher thought, including the condition of suffering and the possibility of experience (Loewy, 1996). To sustain an anencephalic's heart, liver and kidneys without temporarily giving life to the brain stem is a fundamental problem because brain death must occur for organ recovery to begin. Some members of society see an ethical question in the treatment of these infants for the benefit of others. Society's value of these infants may conflict with the values of parents who are willing to donate their infant's organs.

Nurses caring for anencephalic infants often face an ethical dilemma in supporting life-sustaining treatment on behalf of the family or the transplant team. Nurses upholding the principle of non-malfeasance consider these infants the most vulnerable of all. Organ donor transplantation usually requires the donor's consent. Infants cannot consent, and organ transfer or organ recovery must be looked at from a utilitarian approach—the greatest good for the greatest number (Pence, 2000). Additionally, the number of donors is small compared to the cost of procurement and recovery of organs. In a cost-effective health care system, universal access to prenatal care reduces the number of anencephalic births and births of infants with preventable birth defects.

Social Issues Facing Perinatal and Neonatal Nurses
Access to Care and Social Justice

Perinatal nurses often care for pregnant women who present at the hospital in active labor with no prenatal care. Oftentimes, maternal and neonatal complications occur due to a lack of information or late intervention. Regionalization is based on the principle of justice and strives to provide access for all to state-of-the-art perinatal and neonatal technology. Access to care is frustrated at times by the late timing of a pregnant woman's presentation for services. Provider-patient relationships, risk assessment and patient education all contribute to early access to care.

Access to care discussions assume that health care is a right. Internationally, health care and health, itself, are most often believed to be individual rights (Seay, 1996). However, this belief is not universally embraced. For example, libertarians believe that health care is not a right. They believe that forcing a provider to provide health care violates the provider's right to market his/her services for profit.

Many believe that maternal/neonatal health care serves a vulnerable population. From a deontology perspective, a justice-based approach is required, which has prompted social health policy development. Davidoff and Reinecke (1999) proposed drafting the 28th Amendment to the U.S. Constitution to state, "All citizens and other residents of the United States shall have equal access to basic and essential health care" (p. 692). The Emergency Treatment and Active Labor Act (42 U.S.C. Sec. 1395dd, 1990) is a federal mandate for the provision of emergency care services to anyone in need.

There is no comprehensive national approach to prenatal preventative care services. Some states require insurance companies to pay for maternity care and have developed public insurance programs to facilitate access to prenatal care for pregnant women with limited financial resources. However, some women still fail to obtain adequate prenatal care. Factors associated with inadequate prenatal care include poverty, young maternal age, non-married status, lower levels of formal education, negative attitudes toward health care providers, fear and ambivalence regarding pregnancy (Goldenberg, Patterson & Freese, 1992) and involvement in abusive or unsupportive partnerships (Gazmararian, Arrington, Bailey, Schwarz & Koplan, 1999).

Adequate prenatal care has long been associated with improved perinatal health outcomes. After the introduction of organized prenatal care services in the early 20th century, both maternal and infant mortality were markedly reduced (Strong, 2000). Adequate prenatal care begins in the first trimester of pregnancy, with continued and com-

prehensive care throughout the pregnancy. Comprehensive care includes risk assessment, nutritional counseling and patient education (American Academy of Pediatrics & American College of Obstetricians and Gynecologists, 1997) Early prenatal care provides opportunities for health promotion activities, risk assessment and reduction and early diagnosis and intervention. However, comprehensive prenatal care is not the standard. Using a case management approach to prenatal care would ensure the provision of truly comprehensive prenatal care.

Fiscella (1995) examined the evidence for prenatal care as an effective medical intervention for preventing low birthweight. He argued that in light of a questionable, causal relationship between prenatal care and birthweight, as well as inconsistent research results, providers must seek alternative explanations for poor birth outcomes, such as low birthweight. Poor birth outcomes must be viewed contextually as a symptom of broader socioeconomic, cultural and political issues. Contextual factors influencing access to care and the palatability or meaningfulness of prenatal care to the client may be more important to assess than the timing and number of prenatal visits.

The principle of utility generally is upheld by improving access to care. Most health economists believe that prevention is the best medicine for the economy. Health economist Victor Fuchs expressed the need to balance the utilitarian perspective of the greatest good with social justice:

> The problem of inequality [in health status] should be faced head on—in ways that do least damage to the efficient performance of the economy... Paradoxically, the survival of our treasured personal freedom and inde-

A morally good society should ensure access to a basic level of health care.

pendence may depend on our explicitly acknowledging a decent amount of interdependence and responsibility for one another" (Fuchs, 1972, p. 149).

A morally good society should ensure access to a basic level of health care. The current distribution is inequitable. A more efficient and equitable system is needed to assure access and care for all, but not necessarily a wholly egalitarian system (Pence, 2000).

Distributive justice requires major shifts in current therapeutic health care approaches; these changes can only take place in a society where appropriate distribution of resources is a priority. Rationing of services is an essential part of this process. Can society devise a public policy that recognizes a right to care for mothers and infants? A dialogue around access to care is required to establish a distributional system that provides a decent standard of health care to all citizens.

Culturally Competent Care

If, in the interest of social justice, health care is equitably distributed, providers must focus on the unique needs of individuals. A utilitarian perspective asks providers to give the same care to all; however, cultural differences require that care be individually planned and implemented. Individualized care planning is the standard of care (ANA, 1991).

From a cultural perspective, birth is a rite of passage in all cultures. As a key cultural event, birth is imbued with culturally significant ritual and health beliefs. Failure to recognize the cultural significance of birth to a family can cause emotional trauma and set in motion a cascade of culturally constructed threats to the future health of the infant and mother. For example, in some Native American cultures,

traveling at night places an individual at risk from spiritual entities. Pregnant women and infants are at increased risk. What is the significance of a maternal or neonatal transport at night for a family holding such beliefs? Are there rituals that the family would find protective during such a transport?

The fact that an individual health care provider does not share a patient's cultural belief is irrelevant to the needs of the patient, except to remind the provider to move to a heightened level of advocacy for the patient. Cultural competency is the standard of care, yet the diverse nature of society makes it difficult for all health care providers to be cognizant of all cultural beliefs. Clients usually are willing to share their cultural needs with providers who ask about them. Seeking understanding of other views is a foundation of cross-cultural communication.

Cross-cultural communication is complicated by language barrier (Laganá & Gonzalez-Ramirez, in press). To uphold the principle of veracity and, ultimately, the principle of autonomy, qualified medical interpreters must be available. The use of children or other untrained medical interpreters is inappropriate for several reasons. First, for a child, the responsibility of communicating critical information to parents often undermines culturally defined roles of authority and decision making. Secondly, children are legally inappropriate for obtaining informed consent. In addition, the lack of basic medical knowledge in the non-trained interpreter puts the consent process at risk for misinterpretation. Finally, while many cultures actively involve family members in health care decision making, the obligation to respect an individual requires the protection of that individual's privacy. The patient has no opportunity to decide what to tell a family member if the family member serves as the interpreter. In this situation, the patient's right to privacy is violated in exchange for the right to informed consent. This unnecessary ethical dilemma can be avoided with the use of a medical interpreter.

Gender Bias

Some bioethicists believe that a gender bias exists in health care, due in part to the failure of principle-based ethics to incorporate the gender-related experiences of women (Wolf, 1996). Perinatal nurses may have gender bias against fathers, especially fathers who seem less than supportive of their childbearing partners. Gender-specific barriers to ethically competent care have powerful psychosocial, political and cultural affects on the health of childbearing women and their families. As Gilligan (1982) noted, women generally operate from a moral code that is relationship-based. For this reason, it may be difficult for some pregnant women to consider their own welfare separate from those with whom they share strong relationships. Some of the key barriers to upholding the principle of autonomy for pregnant women include culturally prescribed gender roles, ethnicity and race-related outcome disparities, socioeconomic status, domestic violence and inadequate women's health research.

Roles and behaviors for women during childbearing are often prescribed. To deviate from these roles and behaviors places the woman at risk for decreased social support from her group (Laganá, 1996). In many cultures, gender rules assign women to positions of secondary authority for their own self-determination. Women may not feel empowered to make decisions for themselves.

Gender bias in health care research continues to be a problem, although public policy makers are engaging in corrective efforts. Most institutional research review boards consider pregnant women vulnerable because of heightened concern for the non-autonomous fetus. Many researchers avoid research with women of childbearing years.

The American Medical Association's (1991) *Gender Disparities in Clinical Decision Making* reported on data suggesting that a patient's gender plays an inappropriate role in medical decision making. From a public health policy perspective, ethical and legal actions regarding issues such as abortion, surrogate motherhood and maternal-fetal relations must be analyzed in ways that consider potential for gender bias (Wolf, 1996).

Socioeconomic Status

Socioeconomic status plays a role in perinatal health (CDC, 1997). Level of education and financial resources influence the ability for women to make decisions for themselves, as well as their ability to work complex health care systems to their advantage. Ethnic and racial disparity exists in birth outcome for reasons that are unclear.

Domestic Violence

The role of domestic violence in perinatal health must also be considered. Violence against women is primarily partner violence (76 percent) and male perpetrated (Tjaden & Thoennes, 1998). Between 8.8 percent and 29.7 percent of women experience abuse at the hands of their most intimate partners during the perinatal period (Curry, Perrin & Wall, 1998). Women who are abused experience high levels of stress, substance use and social isolation, all of which are associated with poor perinatal outcomes, including preterm birth, low birthweight and perinatal depression (Curry, Perrin &

Gender-specific barriers to ethically competent care have powerful psychosocial, political and cultural affects on the health of childbearing women and their families.

According to the U.S. Census Bureau, in 1996, 44 percent of all children in the United States lived in a non-traditional nuclear family household (without both biological parents and biological siblings.

Wall, 1998). The abused woman and her infant may not be safe for discharge home with an abusive partner, yet disclosure of abuse can present real safety issues. Beneficence and nonmalfeasance are two ethical issues that providers must consider. Safety for the mother and infant are critical. However, poorly managed domestic violence cases can lead to injury or death. Screening for domestic violence should begin in the early prenatal care period to allow for appropriate intervention.

Family-Centered Care

Family is a universal cultural concept. Human beings are born into families and, to varying degrees, continue to function as members of the family group. However, the composition of the family is diverse. The term *postmodern family* (Scanzoni & Marsiglio, 1993) recognizes the profound diversity in family structure and function. According to the U.S. Census Bureau, in 1996, 44 percent of all children in the United States lived in a non-traditional nuclear family household (without both biological parents and biological siblings) (Fields, 2001).

Family-centered maternity care recognizes the integral role of the family in the health care of its members. Family-centered maternity care provides individualized care based on the pregnant woman's psychosocial, cultural, spiritual and physiological needs (Ecenroad, & Zwelling, 2000). Phillips' (1997) principles of family-centered maternity care recognize the mother as the preferred care provider for the infant. Experienced members of the extended family traditionally provide social support and information regarding neonatal and postpartum care. Informed decision making is promoted by optimizing the presence of key familial decision makers. Most perinatal departments have incorporated a family-cen-

tered approach with relaxed visitation rules, the maintenance of infants and mothers as dyads in a rooming-in setting and the inclusion of the woman's partner and other support people.

What happens to a family-centered approach when complications develop? While there may be times when emergent situations require temporary movement away from a family-centered approach, there is little support for this in the literature. In a time of reduced health care resources, providers frequently overlook family members as valuable and resourceful members of the health care team.

Clinical decision making involves informed consent and the application of the principle of autonomy. However, pregnant women and parents often depend on the beliefs and suggestions of significant members of their social networks to make decisions. In the case of neonatal patients, parents are expected to be surrogate decision makers, although research shows that they often feel unprepared for or inadequately supported in this role. Anderson and Hall (1995) described parents reporting difficulty in distinguishing between minor versus major decisions and how they were interrelated. Stress in decision making is increased by the perception of inadequate or inconsistent information, contributing to adversarial relationships between parents and health care providers (Savage, 1997). It may not be clear to parents that signed consent is an act of decision making, rather than a deferral of decision making to the health care team (Miya et al., 1995).

A family-centered approach may be challenging to health care providers when parents are perceived to have abused or neglected their infants (Henry & Purcell, 2000). The most common scenario is the substance-exposed neonate. Most of these neonates go home to their parents. While health care providers may personally have negative feelings toward the parents, it is important to be aware of how those feelings affect a family-centered approach, the promotion of parenting skills and parental/infant attachment.

Finally, while a family-centered approach is the standard of care, it may not meet the individualized needs of parents after delivery (Stainton et al, 1999). The ethical dilemma is that neonatal and perinatal nurses as moral agents have responsibilities for the individual patient and the family. While a family-centered approach upholds the principle of beneficence by promoting naturally occurring support networks, an ongoing assessment of the individual needs of family members upholds the moral obligation to respect the rights of individuals.

Rights of Fathers

Many factors influence the rights of the father as a person and as a surrogate decision-maker. Perhaps most important is the marital status between the childbearing woman and her partner. In the absence of a marital contract, unmarried partners (including same sex partners) lack legal authority to give informed consent for the care of the neonate or the childbearing woman. Once legal paternity is established, some parental rights are provided regarding the neonate. However, durable power of attorney is required for the unmarried partner to actively participate in decision making for the childbearing woman if she is unable to advocate for herself (O'Keefe, 2001).

A review of the literature shows that fathers most often are studied for the affect they have on maternal health outcomes. The limited research that focuses on paternal outcomes indicates that fathers, in a variety of situations in perinatal and neonatal units, often experience stress (Pinelli, 2000; Sydnor-Greenberg & Dokken, 2000; Rimmerman & Sheran, 2001). Table 6 identifies fathers' concerns. Fathers often feel left out (Rimmerman & Sheran, 2001) or ill informed by staff (Chapman, 2000), which may lead to frustration and anger.

Perinatal and neonatal complications often call for ethical decision making regarding treatment plans. Interventions that decrease stress levels in the partners of childbearing women increase the likelihood that partners can participate in a collaborative decision-making process. In addition, perinatal units can facilitate paternal/infant attachment (Resnick, Wattenberg & Brewer, 1994) and promote social support for the childbearing woman by routinely offering to document a legal declaration of paternity.

In the absence of a marital contract, unmarried partners (including same sex partners) lack legal authority to give informed consent for the care of the neonate or the child-bearing woman.

Table 6. Fathers' Concerns
■ Loss of control (Clark & Miles, 1999)
■ Welfare of the infant (Clark & Miles, 1999)
■ Welfare of the partner (Samuelsson, Rådestad & Segesten, 2001)
■ Financial provision for the mother and infant (Hall, 1994; Niska, Lia-Hoagberg & Snyder,1994)
■ Changes in relationships with their partners (Meighan, Davis, Thomas & Droppleman, 1999)
■ Transition into the father role (Dallas, Wilson & Salgado, 2000)
■ Attachment issues (Clark & Miles, 1999)

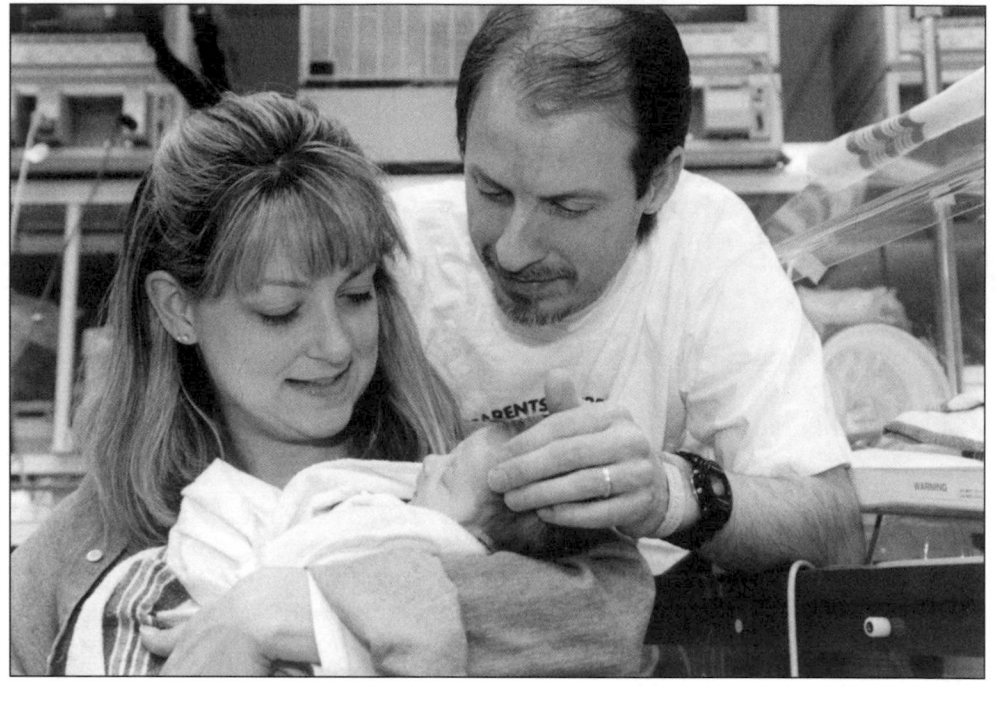

Ethical Decision-Making Models

Nurses as autonomous professionals and key moral agents must provide ethically competent care. They need knowledge of ethical principles and ethical decision-making models to ensure ethical nursing practice (Gaul, 1989). The ANA *Code of Ethics for Nurses with Interpretive Statements* (2001) discusses professional values as a standard for behavior in clinical practice. However, the code, even if incorporated into the nurse's value system, does not provide a systematic framework for ethical decision making. The case study approach is an excellent means for improving this competency.

The Role of Models in Ethical Decision-Making

The use of an ethical decision-making model in a case study format can strengthen the nurse's decision-making abilities. The decision-making framework provided by the models is not meant to solve ethical dilemmas as

they occur in the clinical setting. Many ethical dilemmas develop unexpectedly and frequently require quick decision making. This does not allow the luxury of time to analyze the dilemma. The models, instead, are designed for use with case studies to allow the nurse to utilize ethical principles, analyze value systems and develop an understanding of the nurse as a moral agent and as an active participant in the decision-making process.

As educational tools, case studies should be as comprehensive as possible. Often, however, certain assumptions about the facts of a case must be accepted to move forward in the ethical decision-making process.

The deontological, utilitarian and caring models for ethical decision making use different approaches in the resolution of ethical dilemma. Use of all three models to analyze one case provides a broad view of the dilemma and draws attention to the value systems of those involved in decision making. It is important to reflect on professional values during this process. Analysis of an ethical dilemma from multiple perspectives allows the practicing nurse to develop a broad understanding of values and beliefs that drive ethical decision making in health care settings. The three models are applied to the following case study of Baby K.

Case Study: Baby K

Baby K is a 1-week-old female infant who has been cared for in the neonatal intensive care unit since transfer from a nearby community hospital shortly after birth. She was the product of a full-term pregnancy and an uncomplicated spontaneous vaginal delivery. She is the second infant for her married parents in their late twenties. At 14 hours of age, the infant experienced cardiac arrest while rooming-in with her mother. The infant required full resuscitation and has been maintained on a ventilator since the incident. Providers believe that Baby K's case is near-miss sudden infant death syndrome (SIDS). The neonatologist believes that without the long and vigorous resuscitation effort at the referring hospital, Baby K would not have survived at all.

Baby K has maintained a regular heartbeat but has had no spontaneous movement. Her pupils remain fixed and dilated. EEGs over 2 weeks indicate no regular brain wave activity but have picked up occasional bursts of electrical activity. Because of these bursts of electrical activity, brain death has not been diagnosed. Despite a thorough explanation by the NICU staff that Baby K has sustained irreparable brain damage without hope of recovery, the parents' wishes have remained constant with regard to the infant. They do not want to discontinue life support measures. The parents are aware of cases of miraculous

recovery and want to take all supportive measures to keep Baby K alive. The neonatologist believes the infant to have a poor prognosis, with little chance for survival and no chance of recovery. All members of the health care team believe that to continue life support for Baby K is a futile effort. They believe life support should discontinue, despite the likelihood that Baby K will die shortly thereafter.

The Deontological Ethical Model

In deontology, nurses do not consult their feelings about what to do; instead, they reflect upon their professional duty. In deontology, specific rules guide moral reasoning, and emphasis is on motive, rather than on consequences. Figure 4 identifies steps in the deontological ethical model for the Baby K case.

Step 1. Describe the ethical dilemma. Identification of the dilemma can be a difficult task. In some cases, an ethical dilemma first presents itself as a gnawing feeling that something is wrong with the proposed plan of action. In such a case, it can be helpful to jump ahead to Step 3 of the model and identify ethical rules or principles. The ethical dilemma presented by this case is whether it is ethically correct to maintain Baby K on life support in light of the poor prognosis for recovery.

Step 2. Identify alternative solutions. Once the ethical dilemma has been identified, the nurse should list alternative solutions to the dilemma. In this case, the alternatives are to respect the wishes of the parents and continue life support, to discontinue life support or to set a time limit on continuation of life support.

Step 3. Identify ethical principles.
A. The first principle to consider when an infant or child is involved is that of autonomy. In the health profes-

Figure 4. Laganá-Duderstadt Deontological Ethical Model: Baby K Case Study

Step 1. Describe the ethical dilemma.

Is it ethically correct to maintain Baby K on life support in light of the poor prognosis for recovery?

_____

_____

_____

_____

Step 2. Identify alternative solutions.

1. Continue life support
2. Discontinue life support
3. Set a time limit on continuation of
   life support

_____

_____

_____

_____

_____

3. Identify ethical principles.

a. Autonomy

b. Beneficience

c. Nonmalfeasance

d. Veracity

e. Justice

_____

_____

_____

_____

Step 4.
Analyze alternatives.

Compare solutions
with principles.

One alternative
consistent with
rules or principles

↓

One right action

Alternative consistent
withone rule or principle
conflicts with another

↓

Appeal to higher-level
principle to solve conflict

Step 5. Take action.

Discontinue life support

_____

_____

_____

_____

Adapted from Brody, 1981

sions, this principle is defined as self-determination, but when applied more broadly, it is a general respect for persons and their uniqueness. It is widely accepted that infants and small children lack the cognitive development necessary for self-determination. A surrogate decision-maker usually steps in, most often a parent. The health care provider can, in certain circumstances, serve as a surrogate decision maker, if the courts rule that a parent's decision is not in the best interest of the non-autonomous infant.

B. Perhaps the strongest motivating ethical principle in health care is beneficence. The goal is to intervene in ways that have a beneficial effect on the patient. The principle of beneficence addresses Baby K's best interest. When faced with the inability to do good, as in the case of an irreversible or medically futile situation, the best that health care providers can do is to keep patients from harm.

C. Nonmalfeasance prohibits the intentional infliction of harm, except in situations where that action carries the probability of benefit, such as immunizing a child against disease. The injection may be painful, but the greater benefit of avoiding disease justifies the lesser harm of a painful injection. In addition to asking what benefit continued life support for Baby K will bring, health care providers ask what harm may come from continuation.

D. Providing Baby K's parents with the best available medical judgment, treatment options and associated prognoses adheres to the principle of veracity, the obligation to tell the truth. An assumption of case fact is that this has been done.

E. Providers must consider the principle of justice, the obligation to fairly distribute resources to all members of society. Is it ethically correct to continue to provide health care resources to Baby K?

Step 4. Analyze alternatives.
Once ethical principles have been identified, the next step is to view each alternative individually in light of those principles.

A. The first alternative, to respect the wishes of the parents and continue life support, recognizes the parents as the usual surrogate decision makers for infants and children. Benefit to the infant by following this course must be evaluated, followed by an assessment of what harm might be done by continuing life support.

B. The second alternative is to discontinue life support. This alternative requires overriding the wishes of the parents, possibly through court order. The medical findings suggest that Baby K's condition cannot be corrected by maintaining life support. Therefore, benefit cannot be demonstrated (unless the sanctity of life argument is applied). It is likely, but not certain, that Baby K will die if life support is discontinued. There are many documented cases of persistent vegetative states. Harm (concerning the principle of nonmalfeasance) from continued life support is unclear. Generalized wasting of muscle and bone is associated with prolonged immobility. This can be decreased to some degree by use of passive range of motion and frequent position changes. Perception of pain from medical interventions cannot be determined with any certainty.

Does the expenditure of health care resources for Baby K uphold the principle of justice? Many health care providers would argue that it does not. Discontinuation of life support would free up health care resources to be available for other members of society who might benefit from the receipt of those resources. Discontinuing life support upholds the principle of justice in this case.

C. The third alternative is to set a time limit on continuation of life support. The outcome of this alternative is ultimately the same as discontinuing life support. However, Baby K's parents might be able to spend more time with their daughter, have more time to come to terms with Baby K's condition and be involved in decisions about her care.

Step 5. Take action.
The final step of the deontological model for decision making is to choose the alternative that is supported by ethical principles or rules. Although this sounds simple, it is not. Rules or principles can conflict and, in doing so, one principle must take precedence for a decision to be reached. In this case, veracity conflicts with nonmalfeasance—to uphold the principle of veracity, harm can be caused, while to uphold the principle of nonmalfeasance, the obligation to tell the truth is violated. It is necessary to balance the consequences of violating either of the principles.

In the case of Baby K, the principles of beneficence, nonmalfeasance and veracity are not at risk for violation. The principle of justice, however, is violated when benefits are not distributed evenly throughout society. Providing costly, high-tech medical care to Baby K, who cannot benefit from that care, denies health care resources to another member of society. The most ethically sound solution is to discontinue life support. However, providers must consider the interests of the parents, as this decision usurps their parental rights to act in the best interest of their child. It is the ethical responsibility of the health care provider to take into consideration the harm done to the parents if a decision is made contrary to their wishes.

The Utilitarian Ethical Model
The utilitarian ethical model considers the consequences of the actions taken in ethical decision making. The goal is to choose the action that causes the greatest degree of happiness to the greatest number of involved parties. This model assumes that happiness, or the minimization of unhappiness, is good. Figure 5 identifies steps in the utilitarian ethical model for the Baby K case.

Step 1. Identify the ethical dilemma.
The first step in the use of the utilitarian model, as in the deontological model, is to determine the nature of the ethical problem. The problem in this case is whether to continue Baby K's life support.

Step 2. Define possible actions.
Possible actions are to respect the wishes of the parents to continue life support, to discontinue life support or to set a time limit on continuation of life support.

Step 3. Consider consequences of each possible action.
Action 1, to continue life support, would prolong the physiologic life of Baby K for an undetermined period of time. From the best medical and scientific knowledge available, the prognosis for improvement in the quality of Baby K's life is dismal. Continuation of life support respects the wishes of Baby K's parents, but it does not satisfy

---

Figure 5. Laganá-Duderstadt Utilitarian Ethical Model: Baby K Case Study

---

Step 1. Identify the ethical dilemma.

Is it ethically correct to maintain Baby K on life support in light of the poor prognosis for recovery?

Step 2. Define possible actions.

1. Continue life support

2. Discontinue life support

3. Set a time limit on continuation of life support

Step 3. Consider consequences of each possible action.

1. Prolonged suffering vs. justice; respects parents' wishes

2. Probable death; possible vegetative state; parental involvement

3. Parental acceptance vs. prolonged suffering vs. justice

Step 4. Identify those affected by the decision.

1. Baby K

2. Parents

3. Neonatologist

4. Primary nurse

5. Hospital

6. Society

Step 5. Determine the degree of happiness for each affected party.

See Table 7.

Step 6. Compare happiness scores.

Continue life support = –9

Discontinue life support = +6

Set a time limit on continuation of life support = +9

Adapted from Brody, 1981

Table 7. Scores for Baby K Case					
	Action 1. Continue Life Support		Action 2. Discontinue Life Support		Action 3. Set a Time Limit on Continuation of Life Support
Baby K	Baby K has no cognitive brain function and is unable to perceive happiness.	No score	Baby K has no cognitive brain function and is unable to perceive happiness.	No score	Baby K has no cognitive brain function and is unable to perceive happiness.	No score
Parents	Parents' wishes are respected in the short term, but the prognosis does not change.	++	Action is contrary to the parents' wishes.	– – –	Parental rights are recognized by involving them in decision-making.	– – –
Neonatologist	The neonatologist is unable to help Baby K and feels continuation of life support is futile.	– – –	The neonatologiest feels strongly that life support should be discontinued.	+++	The neonatologist is amenable to this option.	+++
Primary Nurse	The primary nurse feels continuation of life support is futile.	– – –	The primary nurse shares the neonatologist's opinion and is emotionally taxed by caring for Baby K. However, he has also experienced Baby K's parents' grief.	+	The primary nurse finds this action optimal as it addresses the needs and rights of the parents.	+++
Hospital	The hospital may suffer financially from prolonged support to Baby K.	– –	The hospital supports this action for fiscal reasons.	++	The hospital accepts this action.	++
Society	Society continues to pay for Baby K's care. Baby K will never be a contributing member of society.	– – –	Society supports this action.	+++	Society benefits by this action.	+++
Final Happiness Score		+2 −11 −9		+9 −3 +6		+11 −2 +9

the providers' directive to do good. By continuing to provide this technology, they are doing harm to society by wasting precious resources.

Action 2, to discontinue life support, will most probably result in death for Baby K, although a persistent vegetative state cannot be ruled out. This option frees up health care resources for other members of society who are more likely to benefit from those resources. Health care providers, although faced with the loss of a patient, could turn attention to other patients who might benefit from their care giving. The hospital, while possibly saving financial resources (depending on third-party payer reimbursements), must record the death in its perinatal morbidity and mortality count.

Action 3, setting a time limit on continuation of life support, would ultimately have the same outcome as Action 2. Baby K will most likely die or continue in a vegetative state. One consequence of this option is that Baby K's parents could be involved in the decision. In addition, added time assists in addressing outcome uncertainties the parents might have. Finally, time might allow the parents to come to terms emotionally with the reality of Baby K's condition. Resources would continue to be spent until expiration of the time limit.

Step 4. Identify those affected by the decision.
Once possible consequence of the proposed actions is considered, providers must identify those affected by the decision-making process. Baby K is at the center of this group. Others include Baby K's parents, members of the health care team, the hospital and society.

Step 5. Determine the degree of happiness for each affected party
Happiness is symbolized by a plus sign (+), and unhappiness is symbolized by a negative sign (-). Each action has a possible score of three pluses or three negatives for each affected party. This calculation may be offensive to some, this response is reflective of a value system based in deontological thought. However, utilitarian decision making does exist, to some degree, in health care settings.

Some consequences carry heavier weight for certain affected parties. For example, a child's death will be felt most intensely and for a longer period of time by the parents due to the closeness of the bond between parents and their offspring. The death of a child might warrant three negatives (- - -) for the parents, two negatives (- -) for the health care team (to whom death of a patient means failure to do good) and one negative (-) for the hospital that must show a perinatal death in its morbidity and mortality report. Group process facilitates use of the utilitarian ethical model. Providers can role play affected parties to assign pluses and minuses.

Table 7 lists actions and scores for each party in the Baby K case. Action 1, to continue life support, respects the wishes of the parents in the short term, but does not appreciably change the prognosis (+ +). Baby K has no cognitive brain function and is unable to perceive happiness (no score). The health care team is unable to help Baby K and, therefore, feels continuation of life support is futile (- - -). The hospital may suffer financially from prolonged life support to Baby K. Although continuation of life past the perinatal period would result in fewer reported perinatal deaths, this is overshadowed by the hospital's need to survive fiscally (- -). Society would continue to pay for Baby K's care. Even in the event that death does not occur after cessation of life support, Baby K will never be a contributing member of society due to profound brain dysfunction (- - -). By adding up the pluses and minuses, a final happiness score for Action 1 is -6.

Action 2, to discontinue life support, draws a neutral score from Baby K. This action is contrary to the wishes of her parents (- - -). The health care team has some difference of opinion about this action. The neonatologist feels strongly that life support should be discontinued; she feels she has exhausted her ability to give informed consent to the parents and is considering obtaining a court order to discontinue life support (+ + +). The primary nurse shares the neonatologist's opinion of futility in continuing life support. He is emotionally taxed by caring for Baby K. However, he has spent many hours at the bedside with her parents and is saddened by their grief. He feels that court orders are a poor replacement for ongoing and, hopefully, progressive parental informed consent. He feels that, with time, Baby K's parents will accept the prognosis and the medically recommended action (+). For reasons noted in Action 1, the hospital (+ +) and society (+ + +) support this action. The final happiness score for Action 2 is +6.

Action 3, setting a time limit for continuation of life support, recognizes the rights of the parents by involving them in the decision-making process. Additional time may answer parental uncertainties about possible outcomes and facilitate the grieving process. Although the outcome would still be grave, the parents would most likely benefit more from this approach, making the degree of unhappiness less than in Action 2 (- -). The neonatolo-

gist is amenable to this option, as it breaks the stalemate with the parents (+ + +). The primary nurse finds this action optimal as it addresses the needs and rights of the parents (+ + +). The hospital accepts Action 3; acting contrary to the wishes of the parents places the hospital at risk for legal liability. The fiscal loss detracts slightly from the hospital's degree of happiness (+ +). Finally, society benefits from resources freed up by this action (+ + +). The final happiness score for Action 3 is +9.

Step 6. Compare happiness scores. The last step is to compare the happiness scores for each possible action and assign the action with the highest degree of happiness. In this case, setting a time limit on continuation of life support has the highest score at +9.

The Ethical Model of Caring
A criticism of principle-based ethical models is that strict adherence to ethical principles, at times, fails to adequately consider individual needs. In the United States, where law and social custom support individual rights, many believe that failure to recognize individual needs is morally wrong. The decision-making model based on the ethic of caring facilitates moral advocacy for the individual. This model is especially appropriate for those who use a relationship-based approach to decision making (Gilligan, 1982). Figure 6 identifies steps in the ethical model of caring for the Baby K case.

Like the principle-based deontological and utilitarian models, the ethical model of caring encourages in-depth analysis of the ethical dilemma. Unlike the other models, it incorporates contextual forces that affect the patient's (or surrogate decision maker's) decision-making processes.

Step 1. State the ethical dilemma.
This statement is based on the perception of dilemma by the affected individual or, in the case of Baby K, her parents, as her surrogate decision makers, and the health care team. The dilemma is whether to continue Baby K's life support.

Step 2. Describe the context.
Generally, the moral agent must seek additional information to achieve full contextual knowledge. The moral agent interviews Baby K's parents to obtain information about their general health and obstetric history and sociodemographic information.

Baby K's parents are immigrants from an urban center in Somalia where Mr. K worked in the U.S. embassy as a records clerk. Mrs. K is a housewife. Since moving to the United States, Mr. K has worked for a major telecommunications firm. The Ks have excellent health insurance. Both Mr. and Mrs. K have high school educations and speak fluent English. Mr. K has stronger English reading and writing skills than Mrs. K.

Mrs. K has been pregnant five times over the past 7 years. The first three pregnancies ended in first trimester pregnancy losses in Somalia. Two years ago in Washington DC, she delivered a boy at 30 weeks gestation. This infant received state-of-the-art NICU care and survives with mild cerebral palsy.

Step 3. Identify personal relationships.
The next step is to explore the personal relationships involved in the case. Baby K's parents have a traditional, arranged marriage. They have a large extended family, most of whom still live in Somalia. Mrs. K's widowed mother has immigrated to the United States to help raise the K's children. Mrs. K depends a great deal on her

mother's advice. While Mr. K is the predominant communicator with the health care team, he often notes the need to discuss things with his family in Somalia.

Step 4. Analyze the power structure.
Analysis of the Ks' power structure indicates that, although not U.S. citizens, Baby K's parents have permanent residency visas. They have health insurance coverage. However, there is a risk that the medical futility in this case will lead eventually to a discontinuation of benefits. Mr. and Mrs. K have a warm relationship with their obstetrician. However, they have expressed concern to the primary nurse that the neonatologist does not seem to care about their concerns.

Step 5. Assess the degree of informed consent.
An analysis of the degree of informed consent shows that the Ks do not fully understand the irreparable nature of Baby K's brain injury. The medical record shows that the neonatologist documented that full informed consent was provided, including the poor prognosis. The nurse notes that the Ks appear to equate their son's successful NICU experience with a potential positive outcome for Baby K.

Step 6. Identify significant values.
The final step in analysis of this case is to identify value-based ethics that may influence decision making. All people carry beliefs and values regarding human health and life. Values are culturally transmitted and are subject to change as individuals interact with other cultural groups. Values are also influenced by religious beliefs. As traditional Muslims, the Ks believe in the sanctity of life. As urban dwellers, they value the application of technology to manage health problems, and they have reconciled this value with the belief that health care technology is

---

Figure 6. Laganá-Duderstadt Ethical Model of Caring: Baby K Case Study

---

Step 1. State the ethical dilemma.

Is it ethically correct to maintain Baby K on life support in light of the poor prognosis for recovery?

Step 2. Describe the context.

Parents are immigrants from Somalia; they have excellent health insurance; both parents speak fluent English; parents are Muslim; they had three previous pregnancy losses; they have one child with cerebral palsy (CP).

Step 3. Identify personal relationships.

Parents stay in close communication with relatives in Somalia and discuss decisions with them; Mrs. K is dependent on her mother who lives with them to help care for children.

Step 4. Analyze the power structure.

Parents have permanent residency visas; health insurance benefits may discontinue depending on futility of extended care; parents like the obstetrician but aren't comfortable with the neonatologist.

Step 5. Assess degree of informed consent.

Parents don't understand the extent of Baby K's condition; full informed consent was provided; parents believe Baby K will survive NICU experience like their son with CP did.

Step 6. Identify significant values.

Parents believe in the sanctity of life (traditional Muslim belief). They welcome health care technology. Mr. K is primary decision maker, although he relies on his wife's and others' opinions. They believe they have a right to health care in the United States. The health care team agrees Baby K's condition is futile. The nurses think informed consent process should continue due to the parents' belief that Baby K will recover.

Step 7. Make a decision.

Ensure that informed consent has been given and continue process until conditions change.

---

provided by Allah. As a Muslim woman, Mrs. K is influenced by gender role that places her husband as the primary decision maker. However, the Ks have demonstrated a somewhat egalitarian relationship at Baby K's bedside, in which Mr. K has elicited his wife's and mother's-in-law opinions. As immigrants and Muslims, they perceive that they have experienced discrimination since arriving in the United States. But, as permanent U.S. residents, they are adamant that they and their children have the same rights to health care as other Americans. The neonatologist believes that continuation of care for Baby K in the face of medical futility violates the principle of utility. The nurses caring for Baby K agree with the neonatologist, but they temper this agreement with an obligation to care for the family. This obligation involves the extended family in decision making. The nurses also believe that the informed consent process needs to continue, as there is a discrepancy between the neonatologist's written prognosis and the parents' observed hopefulness for Baby K's recovery.

Step 7. Make a decision.
The result of this decision-making process may not be an immediate life or death decision; it may be to ensure that full, informed consent has been given and cycling back through the model's steps as conditions change and new case facts emerge. The ethic of caring is an ongoing process, assisting and supporting Baby K's parents as they and the health care team move toward resolution.

Summary
Technological and social issues affecting the health of pregnant women and their infants are complex. This complexity requires a comprehensive assessment of ethical issues involved. Nurses as autonomous professionals and key moral agents are required to provide ethically competent care. The case study approach is an excellent means for improving this competency. The deontological, utilitarian and ethical caring models for decision making use different approaches in the resolution of ethical dilemma. Use of all three models to analyze one case provides a broader view of the dilemma and draws attention to the value systems of those involved in ethical decision making. It is important to reflect on professional values during this process, especially respect for persons as individuals and as members of a broader family group, community and society.

Application of ethical theory to actual clinical practice is, at times, challenging. The following case studies will help the practicing perinatal or neonatal nurse recognize how ethical theory translates to ethical practice.

The decision-making models presented in this module are designed for use in a case study format. Applying the models to the following case studies will increase the nurse's awareness of the ethical decision-making process and help the nurse understand how philosophical approach and personal beliefs influence thinking about ethical dilemma.

The application of ethically complex cases to one of the three decision-making models can be approached individually or in a group format. If used in a group study, the facilitator may want to break into small groups by ethical approach—deontological, utilitarian and ethic of care—to analyze a single case. Each break-out group should discuss the case, apply the decision-making model and share the process and results with the larger group.

As case studies are limited by the details provided, it is appropriate to choose one person in the group to provide additional case history, if needed. This allows the group to move past sticking places in the discussion. However, if this approach is used, the chosen person should serve as a facilitator only and not participate in the decision-making process.

Case #1. The Fetus on the Edge of Viability

Ann is a labor and delivery nurse in a 600-bed university hospital. She is assigned to the new admission, a laboring woman who is a Gravida 3 Para 0 SAB 2. She is spontaneously aborting a 21- to 23-week fetus. Dates of gestation are estimated, and the fetus is expected to weigh <500 g.

Ann asks if the delivery should take place in the delivery room and if resuscitation measures are to be taken. She knows that resuscitation equipment is not readily available in the labor rooms. She is told to let the woman deliver in bed in the labor room and to call the pediatrician if the infant shows signs of life. Ann hears the woman calling for help. She enters the room in time to catch the baby being delivered. The physician on duty follows and notes that the infant has a heart rate and is grunting. The pediatrician is paged to the labor room.

The pediatric resident arrives within minutes. The infant is wrapped in a blanket and is transported immediately to the intensive care nursery. The infant weighs approximately 700 g, has a weak heart rate of 60 and no spontaneous respirations. The pediatrician elicits help from Ann to continue resuscitation. Ann questions the pediatrician's request for help in light of the prognosis for this neonate.

Case #2. The Failed Home Delivery

Susan Smith presents to the labor and delivery unit of a community hospital at 2:40 a.m. in a small, West coast town. She is full term. She is accompanied by her lay midwife and her husband. She has been laboring at home for 2 days. The midwife reports that Ms. Smith's membranes ruptured 18 hours earlier with lightly meconium-stained amniotic fluid. She convinced the couple to go to the hospital after she heard several decelerations on auscultation. On admit, Ms. Smith's cervix is completely dilated; the midwife says it has been dilated for 3 hours and that Ms. Smith has pushed for most of the 3 hours. A large caput is noted, but the station of the presenting part can not be determined.

The labor and delivery nurse places Ms. Smith on continuous electronic fetal monitoring. The nurse notes the FHR to be without variability and positive for late decelerations that do not resolve with IV fluids, oxygen or maternal position changes. Ms. Smith does not have a regular obstetrician, so an in-house obstetrician sees her. She tells Ms. Smith that she needs an immediate cesarean delivery. Mrs. Smith agrees to the c-section, but Mr. Smith protests; it takes a half hour to convince him to support his wife in her decision.

Anesthesia is called in, and the baby is delivered about 25 minutes after Ms. Smith gives informed consent for the cesarean delivery. The infant boy weighs 4,200 g and needs vigorous resuscitation with APGAR scores of 1, 4, and 9 at 1, 5 and 10 minutes, respectively. The infant begins seizures shortly after birth and is transported to the regional medical referral center for intensive care. The infant is ultimately diagnosed with cerebral palsy.

At the change of shift report, the admitting nurse expresses concern to the other nurses that the infant's condition is probably related to the long labor and delay in obtaining medical care. A short discussion ensues between the nurses about whether the Smiths should be informed of this concern. Three days later, the obstetrician shares with the Smiths a similar view about the long labor and delay in care. The discussion, however, is not clearly documented in the medical record. A malpractice claim is eventually filed by the Smiths against the lay midwife.

Case #3. The Anencephalic Infant

Laura Campo did not have medical insurance and did not seek prenatal care until the 24th week of pregnancy. She learned when she was 8 months pregnant that her baby was anencephalic. Because the diagnosis was made so late in pregnancy, she could not have an abortion. Ms. Campo heard about organ donation from anencephalic infants on a talk show. She decided to bring the fetus to term to donate the organs. Because an anencephalic infant often has a swollen head, vaginal delivery risks fetal demise and damage to organs for transplantation. Ms. Campo understood that she would need a cesarean delivery. Baby Theresa was born on March 21, 1992 in Fort Lauderdale, Florida.

Providers expected Baby Theresa to die within minutes after birth, but she did not. Baby Theresa had to be declared brain dead before her organs could be donated. Her parents asked that she be declared brain dead. However, Baby Theresa did not meet the criteria for brain death under Florida law, and the neonatologist refused to remove the organs (Pence, 2000). Pictures of Baby Theresa showing a beautiful baby girl wearing a pink knitted cap that covered the top half of her head were distributed to the press. Underneath the cap were no skin, no skull and no cerebrum.

The couple appealed to the Florida circuit court to rule that Baby Theresa was dead. The judge ruled that she was unable to authorize taking Baby Theresa's life to save another. The couple appealed to the Florida District Court of Appeals, which affirmed the circuit court's decision. As the case grew in publicity, the parents appealed to the Florida Supreme Court. The Florida Supreme Court lacked constitutional authority to hear the case because the District Court of Appeals had ruled that it was not of "great public importance" (Pence, 2000).

On March 29, Baby Theresa's organs began to fail. By the time the respirator was removed, the organs were unusable for transplantation. Baby Theresa died on March 30, and her organs were useless for transplantation.

Case #4. The Donor Sibling
In 1991, Abe and Mary Alaya's daughter Anissa is diagnosed with a rare form of leukemia. The only possibility for a cure is a bone marrow transplant. However, the Alayas cannot find a suitable donor. As a last effort, the Alayas decide to conceive another child, with the hope that the offspring will be a good match with Anissa. Abe has his vasectomy reversed, and Mrs. Alaya conceives and has a baby girl. Against 4 to 1 odds, Anissa's sister is a match. The bone marrow transplant is successful, and Anissa (and her baby sister) survives.

Case #5. Experimental Fetal Surgery
Grace is a full-term infant born with hypoplastic left heart. At birth, she is medically transported across state borders to the NICU at a large tertiary center for a complex cardiac procedure. This procedure has been attempted only a handful of times on small infants, and Grace is one of the smallest. Following the procedure, Grace is placed on a left ventricular assist device (LVAD) after attempts to wean her off cardiopulmonary bypass are unsuccessful. Because the procedure to repair her cardiac defect is experimental, her sternal bone is left open and the area closed by silastic patch. She is maintained on multiple vasoactive drugs and ventilation and receives exceedingly complex medical care. Grace is eventually weaned and decannulated from the LVAD. Her postoperative course is not clear, however, as the staged cardiac repair is experimental.

Complications eventually take hold. Grace develops a clot in her heart. The care team begins a tissue plasminogen activator (TPA), which makes her bleed excessively and necessitates complete replacement of her circulating volume multiple times a day for several days. During this time, Grace remains responsive, even though she is on analgesic and sedative infusions. Nursing care for her and her family is emotionally challenging. Eventually the clot dissolves, and she does not suffer many of the complications associated with multiple total blood volume exchanges. At this point, her sternum has been open for a month, and the surgical team feels it should attempt chest closure. Due to the size of Grace's heart, the team is only able to get two-thirds of the area closed without compromising Grace's tenuous hemodynamics. The lower third remains open, and the plan is to close this area by granulation. This is an unconventional treatment plan and controversial among much of the staff.

Case #6. Discharge to the Unsafe Home

Thirty-four-year-old Susan is well known to the labor and delivery staff. She is a recovered methamphetamine user who lost custody of her first three children shortly after their births because of positive drug screens.

Two years ago, Susan decided she wanted to have a healthy life and regain custody of her children. She divorced her husband, a convicted and incarcerated drug dealer. She enrolled in a 6-month residential rehabilitation program on court order and was drug-free for more than 18 months. She also took parenting classes and was assigned a community-based lay counselor. She met her new boyfriend, Joe, a recovering drug user, at a counseling session. They moved in together, and a few months later, Susan was pregnant. She was determined to keep this child. She volunteered for drug screening throughout her pregnancy. However, during the pregnancy, Joe began using drugs again, was more irritable than usual and hit Susan twice.

Susan's daughter Silvia is born drug-free. Breastfeeding is well established, and Susan demonstrates strong infant care skills and maternal/infant attachment. Joe is not present for Silvia's birth, but he does visit for several hours after. He is much younger than Susan, and Silvia is his first child. Silvia is released home with her mother.

The postpartum nurse worries as she does discharge planning. First, the nurse is concerned for Susan's and Silvia's safety due to Joe's violent behavior and renewed drug use. Secondly, the nurse is worried that Susan will relapse into drug use and that Silvia might be neglected or even abused.

The following discussion items aid the learner in applying concepts presented in this module.

1. Informed consent aims to uphold the principle of autonomy and the right to self-determination. Within your group, explore occurrences in which the level of informed consent seemed inadequate to you. What other ethical principles came into play?

2. The use of technology requires strong nursing skills. What ethical approach would you take if asked to use a technology for which you lack skills?

Perinatal and Neonatal Ethics: Facing Contemporary Challenges

To receive continuing education credit for completion of this module via independent study, record answers to the following questions on the Independent Study Application and submit it to March of Dimes for grading. Submission instructions are listed on the application.

1. An ethical dilemma unique to perinatal nursing is the:
   A. Risk of malfeasance
   B. Intensive use of technology
   C. Shortage of health care resources
   D. Innate conflict between maternal and fetal rights

2. A nurse's individual value development is essential for:
   A. Making decisions that influence society
   B. Participating in ethical decision making
   C. Advocating ethical courses of action that follow the rules
   D. Promoting the rights of the fetus from the point of conception

3. Which nursing situation reflects the concept of veracity?
   A. Reviewing the side effects associated with tocolytics
   B. Supporting the patient's choice of medical intervention
   C. Ensuring that both fetal and maternal rights are considered
   D. Guaranteeing that a high-risk mother delivers in a Level III perinatal care facility

4. The American Nurses Association *Code of Ethics for Nurses* directs nurses to provide patient care that is:
   A. Curative
   B. Utilitarian
   C. Respectful
   D. Autonomous

5. When assessing if a procedural risk to a mother or fetus is justified, the ethical principle underlying the dilemma is:
   A. Nonmaleficence
   B. Informed consent
   C. Self-determination
   D. Respect for the fetus

6. The major conceptual foundation of deontology is that people have a specific duty to:
   A. Maximize good within a society
   B. Do what is right for the individual
   C. Bend the rules when it will help a patient
   D. Consider the consequences of decisions in relation to others

7. In which situation is the ethical concept of justice violated?
   A. The promotion of perinatal service regionalization
   B. The retrieval and storage of cord blood from a newborn
   C. An insurance company's refusal to pay for in vitro fertilization
   D. A court-ordered obstetric treatment program for a pregnant woman who abuses drugs

8. Level II, Conventional Morality, in Kohlberg's Moral Development Model reflects the moral philosophy that doing right is related to:
   A. Justice
   B. What is fair
   C. Fulfilling one's role
   D. Good for the greatest number

9. To best help parents confronted with a perinatal moral dilemma, the nurse must approach the situation with:
   A. Good judgment
   B. Unwavering values
   C. A personal moral philosophy
   D. A decision-making framework

10. The parents of a fetus with multiple anomalies decide to have an abortion. They state that the child would have no quality of life and would negatively affect their ability to provide for their other children. The parents' decision reflects the ethical concepts associated with:
    1. Deontology
    2. Utilitarianism
    3. Gilligan's Theory
    4. Kohlberg's Theory

11. The word most closely associated with the ethic of caring is:
    A. Veracity
    B. Empathy
    C. Dilemma
    D. Negotiation

12. Which best reflects a relationship to the technological imperative identified by Vimpani?
    A. Paternalism infringing on patient autonomy
    B. Distributive justice ensuring equal accessibility to care
    C. Health care practices addressing the needs of both mother and fetus
    D. Medical initiatives promoting a reduction in infant mortality in the United States

13. A feeling basic to the underlying etiology of moral distress is:
    A. Anger
    B. Sorrow
    C. Hopelessness
    D. Powerlessness

14. Which clinical situation best reflects support of the ethical principle of beneficence?
    A. Signing an informed consent
    B. Disclosing the potential negative outcomes of therapy
    C. Providing intensive care to a very-low-birthweight infant
    D. Ensuring that pregnant women have access to prenatal care

15. Tiedge's Moral Action Model presents a framework for ethical decision making to:
    A. Decrease the incidence of ethical dilemmas
    B. Simplify the ethical decision-making process
    C. Enable nurses to make ethically sound decisions for patients
    D. Promote active participation in the decision-making process

Perinatal and Neonatal Ethics: Facing Contemporary Challenges

To receive continuing education credit for registered nurses and certified nurse-midwives via independent study of *Perinatal and Neonatal Ethics: Facing Contemporary Challenges*:

1. Complete the registration information.
2. Legibly write the letter of the answer for each question in the spaces provided.
3. Sign and date the application.
4. Return the application and the tear-out self-mailer evaluation to: Nursing Modules, March of Dimes, 1275 Mamaroneck Avenue, White Plains, NY 10605.

The March of Dimes will notify you of your results within 8 weeks of receiving your completed test. If you receive a passing score (70 percent), you will receive a certificate of completion indicating the amount of continuing education earned. If your score is less than 70 percent, you will be given a second opportunity to pass the test.

This continuing education activity was approved by the New York State Nurses Association, an accredited approver by the American Nurses Credentialing Center's Commission on Accreditation. **It has been approved for 5.22 contact hours for registered nurses.**

The March of Dimes is also approved as a continuing education provider by the State of California Board of Registered Nursing, Provider #CEP-111444.

This module is also approved for .4 continuing education units (CEUs) for certified nurse-midwives (CNMs) by the American College of Nurse-Midwives (ACNM) (program #2003/085). ACNM approval expires 10/24/05. CNMs should verify the module's approval status at marchofdimes.com/professionals if the module is used after the expiration date.

REGISTRATION INFORMATION

Name _____

Credentials _____

Address _____

City _____ State _____ ZIP _____

Telephone _____ Fax _____

E-mail _____

INDEPENDENT STUDY TEST ANSWERS

1. _____	5. _____	9. _____	13. _____
2. _____	6. _____	10. _____	14. _____
3. _____	7. _____	11. _____	15. _____
4. _____	8. _____	12. _____	

Signature _____ Date _____

CHECKLIST FOR MAILING

☐ Completed (and signed) application
☐ Completed evaluation

Aaronson, L. & Macnee, C. (1989). Tobacco, alcohol and caffeine use during pregnancy. *JOGNN*, *18*(4), 279-287.

Agency for Health Care Research and Quality. (2000). Management of preterm labor. Summary, evidence report/technology assessment number 18. *Agency for Healthcare Research and Quality Pub. No. 01E020*. Rockville, MD: Author.

Alexander, B. (2001). (You)2 .*Wired*. February, 120-135.

Allmark, P. (1995). Can there be an ethics of care? *Journal of Medical Ethics, 21*, 19-24.

American Academy of Pediatrics (AAP) and American College of Obstetricians and Gynecologists (ACOG). (1997). *Guidelines for perinatal care* (4th ed.). Elk Grove Village, IL: AAP.

American College of Obstetricians and Gynecologists (ACOG). (2001). Assessment of risk factors for preterm birth. Clinical management guidelines for obstetricians-gynecologists. ACOG Practice Bulletin, No. 31. *Obstetrics and Gynecology, 98*(4), 709-716.

American College of Obstetricians and Gynecologists (ACOG). (1987a). *Patient choice: Maternal-fetal conflict*. Washington, DC: Author.

American College of Obstetricians and Gynecologists (ACOG). (1987b). *Statement on court-ordered obstetrical interventions*. Washington, DC: Author.

American Medical Association. (1991). Gender disparities in clinical decision making. *JAMA, 266*, 559-562.

American Nurses Association (ANA). (2001). *Code of ethics for nurses with interpretive statements*. [Online]. Available: www.nursingworld.org/ethics/ecode.htm

American Nurses Association (ANA). (1991). *Position paper on cultural diversity in nursing practice*. Kansas City, MO: Author.

American Nurses Association (ANA). (2000). *Position statement: Human cloning by means of blastomere splitting and nuclear transplantation*. Washington, DC: Author.

American Society for Reproductive Medicine (ASRM). (2000a). Financial incentives in recruitment of oocyte donors. *Fertility and Sterility, 74*(2), 216-220.

American Society for Reproductive Medicine (ASRM). (2000b). Human somatic cell nuclear transfer (cloning). *Fertility and Sterility, 74*(5), 873-876.

American Society for Reproductive Medicine (ASRM). (2001). Preconception gender selection for nonmedical reasons. *Fertility and Sterility, 75*(5), 861-864.

American Society for Reproductive Medicine (ASRM). (1999). Preimplantation genetic diagnosis and sex selection. *Fertility and Sterility, 72*(4), 595-598.

Anderson, B. & Hall, B. (1995). Parents' perceptions of decision-making for children. *J Law Med Ethics, 23*(1), 15-9.

Andre, J. (1998). Learning from nursing. *Med Human Ret*, Winter(1), 3-7.

Annas, G. (1982). Forced Cesareans: The most unkindest cut of all. *The Hastings Report, 12*(3), 16-17, 45.

Annas, G. (1998). The shadowlands: Secrets, lies, and assisted reproduction. *New England Journal of Medicine, 339*(13), 935-939.

Antoine, M. (1989). Court-ordered medical treatment. *California Nursing Review*, September/October, 20-23.

Association of Women's Health, Obstetric and Neonatal Nursing (AWHONN). (2000). *Infertility treatment issue: Infertility treatment as a covered health insurance benefit.* Washington, DC: Author.

Bandman, E. & Bandman, B. (1995). *Nursing ethics through the lifespan* (3rd ed.). Stamford, CT: Appleton & Lange.

Beauchamp, T.L. & Childress, J.F. (1994). *Principles of biomedical ethics* (4th ed.). New York: Oxford University Press.

Beck, C. (1996a). A meta-analysis of predictors of postpartum depression. *Nursing Research, 45*, 297-303.

Beck, C. (1996b). Postpartum depressed mothers' experiences interacting with their children. *Nursing Research, 45*, 98-104.

Behnke, M., Eyler, F., Conlon, M., Casanova, O. & Woods, N. (1997). How fetal cocaine exposure increases neonatal hospital costs. *Pediatrics 99*(2), 204-208.

Berkowitz, R., Lynch, L., Chitkara, U., Wilkins, I.A., Mehalek, K.E. & Alvarez, E. (1988). Selective reduction of multifetal pregnancies in the first trimester. *New England Journal of Medicine, 318*, 1043-1047.

Beski, S., Gorgy, A., Venka, G., Craft, I.L. & Edmonds, K. (2000). Gestational surrogacy: A feasible option for patients with Rokitansky Syndrome. *Human Reproduction, 15*(11), 2326-2328.

Bowers, N. (1998). The multiple birth explosion: Implications for nursing practice. *JOGNN, 27*(3), 302-310.

Brody, H. (1981). *Ethical decisions in medicine* (2nd ed.). Boston: Little, Brown & Company.

Buzzanca v. Buzzanca, 61 Cal. App. 4th 1410, 1998.

Caffrey, R.A. & Caffrey, P.A. (1994). Nursing: caring or codependency? *Nursing Forum, 29*(1), 12-17.

Cahill, L. (1988). The ethics of surrogate motherhood: Biology, freedom and moral obligation. *Law, Medicine & Healthcare, 16*(1), 65-71.

Cameron, A. (1981). *Daughters of copper woman.* Vancouver, BC: Gang Press.

Carrico, J. (2001). The Human Genome Project: An update. *Medscape Pharmacology Journal. 3*(3), 1-5.

Carse, A.L. (1991). The "voice of care": Implications for bioethical education. *The Journal of Medicine and Philosophy, 16,* 5-28.

Centers for Disease Control and Prevention (CDC). (1999a). *1997 assisted reproductive technology success rates. National summary and fertility clinic reports.* Atlanta, GA: Author.

Centers for Disease Control and Prevention (CDC). (2000a). *1998 assisted reproductive technology success rates: National summary and fertility clinic reports.* Atlanta, GA: Author.

Centers for Disease Control and Prevention (CDC). 2002. Alcohol use among women of childbearing age—United States, 1991-1995. *Morbidity and Mortality Weekly Report, 51*(13), 273-76.

Centers for Disease Control and Prevention (CDC). (2000b). Contribution of assisted reproductive technology and ovulation-inducing drugs to triplet and higher-order multiple births—United States, 1980-1997. *MMWR, 49*(24), 535-538.

Centers for Disease Control and Prevention (CDC). (1997). *Fertility, family planning and women's health: New data from the 1995 National Survey of Family Growth.* Atlanta, GA: Author.

Centers for Disease Control and Prevention (CDC). (1995). Medical-care expenditures attributable to cigarette smoking during pregnancy—United States, 1995. *MMWR, 46*(44), 1048-1050.

Centers for Disease Control and Prevention (CDC). (1999b). Preterm singleton births—United States, 1989-1996. *MMWR, 48*(9), 185-189.

Centers for Disease Control and Prevention (CDC). 2003. *State prenatal smoking databook, 1999.* [Online]. Available: http://www.cdc.gov/nccdphp/drh/PrenatalSmkbk

Chapman, L. (2000). Expectant fathers and labor epidurals. *MCN, The American Journal of Maternal-Child Nursing, 25*(3), 133-138.

Chavkin, W. (1992). Women and fetus: The social construction of conflict. In C. Feinman (Ed.), *The Criminalization of a Woman's Body.* New York: Harrington Park Press.

Chervenak, F. & McCullough, L. (1985). Perinatal ethics: A practical method of analysis of obligations to mother and fetus. *Obstetrics and Gynecology, 66*(3), 442-446.

Child Abuse Prevention and Treatment Act. 42 U.S.C. 1983.

Childress, J. (1990). The place of autonomy in bioethics. *The Hastings Center Report, 14*(5), 32-35.

Clark, S.M. & Miles, M.S. (1999). Conflicting responses: The experiences of fathers of infants diagnosed with severe congenital heart disease. *Journal of the Society of Pediatric Nurses, 4*(1), 7-14.

Clayton, E., Steinberg, K., Khoury, M., Thomson, E., Andrews, L., Kahn, M., Kopelman, L. & Weiss, J. (1995). Informed consent for genetic research on stored tissue samples. *JAMA, 274*(22), 1786-1792.

Cordero, L., Backes, C. & Zuspan, F. (1982). Very-low-birthweight infant: Influence of place of birth on survival. *American Journal of Obstetrics and Gynecology, 143*, 533-537.

Curry, M., Perrin, N. & Wall, E. (1998). Effects of abuse on maternal complications and birthweight in adult and adolescent women. *Obstetrics and Gynecology, 92*(4), 530-534.

Dallas, C., Wilson, T. & Salgado, V. (2000). Gender differences in teen parents' perceptions of parental responsibilities. *Public Health Nursing, 17*(6), 423-433.

Davidoff, F. & Reinecke, R. (1999). The 28th Amendment. *Annals of Internal Medicine, 130*(8), 692-694.

Davis, A.J. & Aroskar, M.A. (1983). *Ethical dilemmas and nursing practice* (2nd ed.). Norwalk, CT: Appleton-Crofts.

Doroshow, R.W., Hodgman, J.E., Pomerance, J.J., Ross, J.W., Michel, V.J., Luckett, P.M. & Shaw, A. (2000). Treatment decisions for newborns at the threshold of viability: An ethical dilemma. *Journal of Perinatology, 20*, 379-383.

Drug found in babies, and mother is guilty. (1989, July 14). *The New York Times*, p. A10.

Dunham, C. (1991). Mamatoto: A Celebration of Birth. New York: Penguin Books.

Emergency Treatment and Active Labor Act. 42 U.S.C. Sec. 1395dd. 1990.

Ecenroad, D. & Zwelling, E. (2000). A journey to family-centered maternity care. *MCN, The American Journal of Maternal-Child Nursing, 25*(4), 178-186.

Falk Rafael, A. (1996). Power and caring: A dialectic in nursing. *Advances in Nursing Science, 19*(1), 3-17.

Federal Register. (1985). Public Law 98-457.

Fields, J. (2001). Living arrangements of children: Household economic studies, 1996. *Current Population Reports*, P70-74. Washington DC: U.S. Census Bureau.

Finkelstein, N. (1994). Treatment issues for alcohol- and drug-dependent pregnant and parenting women. *Health and Social Work, 19*, 7-15.

Fiscella, K. (1995). Does prenatal care improve birth outcomes? A critical review. *Obstetrics and Gynecology, 85*(3), 468-479.

Fletcher, J.C. (1979). *Humanhood: Essays in biomedical ethics*. Buffalo: Prometheus Books.

Flynn, K. (1999). Preterm labor and premature rupture of membranes. In L. Mandeville & N. Troiano (Eds.), *AWHONN High-risk and Critical Care Intrapartum Nursing* (2nd ed.). Philadelphia: Lippincott.

Four boys, three girls! (November 19, 1997), *The Des Moines Register*, p. 1.

Francis, G. & Nosek, J. (1988). Ethical considerations in contemporary reproductive technologies. *Journal of Perinatal and Neonatal Nursing, 1*(3), 37-48.

Francoeur, R. (1983). *Biomedical ethics: A guide to decision-making*. New York: John Wiley & Sons.

Francoeur, R. (1985). From then to now: The evolution of bioethical decision-making in perinatal intensive care. In C. Harris & F. Snowden (Eds.), *Bioethical Frontiers in Perinatal Intensive Care*. Natchitoches, LA: Northwestern State University Press.

Frankena, W.K. (1973). *Ethics* (2nd ed.). Englewood Cliffs, NJ: Prentice-Hall.

Freda, M.C. & Patterson, E.T. (2004). *Preterm labor: Prevention and nursing management* (3rd ed.). White Plains, NY: March of Dimes.

Fuchs, V. (1972). *Who shall live?* New York: Basic Books, Inc.

Gaul, A. (1989). Ethics content in baccalaureate degree curricula. *Nursing Clinics of North America, 24*(2), 475-483.

Gazmararian, J., Arrington, T., Bailey, C., Schwarz, K. & Koplan, J. (1999). Prenatal care for low-income women enrolled in a managed-care organization. *Obstetrics and Gynecology, 94*(2), 177-185.

Gilligan, C. (1982). *In a different voice*. Cambridge, MA: Harvard University Press.

Goepfert, A.R., Goldenberg, R.L., Mercer, B., Iams, J., Meis, P., Moawad, A., Thom, E., VanDorsten, J.P., Caritis, S.N., Thurnau, G., Miodovnik, M., Dombrowski, M., Roberts, J.M. & McNellis, D. (2000). The preterm prediction study: Quantitative fetal fibronectin values and the prediction of spontaneous preterm birth. *American Journal of Obstetrics and Gynecology, 183*(6), 1480-1483.

Goldenberg, R., Patterson, E. & Freese, M. (1992). Maternal demographics, situational, and psychosocial factors and their relationship to enrollment in prenatal care: A review of the literature. *Women & Health, 19*(2-3), 133-151.

Greenlee, S. (2000). Dolly's legacy to human cloning: International legal responses and potential human rights violations. *Wisconsin University Law Journal, 18*, 537.

Hall, W. (1994). New fatherhood: Myths and realities. *Public Health Nursing, 11*, 219-228.

Harris, L. (2000). Rethinking maternal-fetal conflict: Gender and equality in perinatal ethics. *Obstetrics and Gynecology, 96*(5, Pt.1), 786-791.

Hazebroek, F.W., Smeets, R.M., Bos, A.P., Owens, C., Tibboel, D. & Molenaar, J.C. (1996). Staff attitudes toward continuation of life-support in newborns with major congenital anomalies. *European Journal of Pediatrics, 155*(9), 783-786.

Held, V. (1995). *Justice and care: Essential readings in feminist ethics.* Boulder, CO: Westview Press, Inc.

Henry, J. & Purcell, R. (2000). Exploring the tensions being family centered with parents who abuse/neglect their children. Infant-Toddler Intervention: *The Transdisciplinary Journal, 10*(4), 275-285.

Hopkins, P. (1998). Bad copies: How popular media represent cloning as an ethical problem. *Hastings Center Report, March/April,* 6-13.

Hornstra, D. (1998). A realistic approach to maternal-fetal conflict. *Hastings Center Report, September/October,* 7-12.

Hughes, P., Coletti, S., Neri, R., Urmann, C., Stahl, S., Sicilian, D. & Anthony, J. (1995). Retaining cocaine-abusing women in a therapeutic community: The effect of a child live-in program. *American Journal of Public Health, 85,* 1149-1152.

Jameson, A.J. (1993). Dilemmas of moral distress: Moral responsibility and nursing practice. *AWHONN's Clinical Issues, 4*(4), 542-551.

Jefferson v. Griffin Spalding City Hospital. 274 S.E., 2nd 457, GA, 1981.

Kass v. Kass. 235 A.D. 2nd 150, 663 N.Y. S. 2nd 581(App. Div. 2nd Dept. 1997).

Kearney, M.H. (1997). Drug treatment for women: Traditional models and new directions. *JOGNN, 26*(4):459-68.

King, N. (1991). Maternal-fetal conflicts: Ethical and legal implications for nurse-midwives. *Journal of Nurse-Midwifery, 36*(6), 361-365.

Kohlberg, L. (1984). *The psychology of moral development: The nature of validity of moral stages.* San Francisco: Harper & Row.

Klotzko, A.J. (1998). Medical miracle or medical mischief? The saga of the McCaughey septuplets. *Hastings Center Report, 28*(3), 5-8.

Kolder, V., Gallagher, J. & Parsons, M. (1987). Court-ordered obstetrical interventions. *New England Journal of Medicine, 316*(19), 1192-1196.

Kopelman, L.M., Irons, T.G. & Kopelman, A.E. (1988). Neonatologists judge the "Baby Doe" regulations. *New England Journal of Medicine, 318,* 677-683.

Laganá, K. (1994). Upfront: Women, healing and the feminine perspective. *AWHONN: Women's Health Nursing Scan, 8*(5), 1-2.

Laganá. K. (1996). Preventing low birthweight: Cultural influences on Mexican immigrant and Mexican American prenatal care. A community study. *Dissertation Abstracts International.* 57/06B.

Laganá, K. (2000). The "right" to a caring relationship: Law and ethic of care. *Journal of Perinatal & Neonatal Nursing, 14*(2), 12-24.

REFERENCES

Laganá, K. & Gonzalez-Ramirez, L. (in press). Mexican Americans. In P. St. Hill, J. Lipson & A. Meleis (Eds.), *Caring for Women Cross-Culturally: A Portable Guide*. Philadelphia: F.A. Davis.

Lam, F. (1991). Miniature pump infusion of terbutaline: An option in preterm labor. *Contemporary Ob/Gyn, 33*(1), 52-70.

Larkin, M. (2000). Curb costs of egg donation, urge U.S. specialists. *The Lancet, 356*(9229), 569.

Lewit, E., Baker, L., Corman, H. & Shiono, P. (1995). The direct cost of low birth weight. *The Future of Children, 5*(1), 35-56.

Lieberman, E., Gremy, I., Lang, J. & Cohen, A. (1994). Low birthweight at term and the timing of fetal exposure to maternal smoking. *American Journal of Public Health, 84*(7), 1127-1131.

Loewy, E.H. (1995). Care ethics: A concept in search of a framework. *Cambridge Quarterly of Healthcare Ethics, 4*, 56-63.

Loewy, E.H. (1996). *Textbook of healthcare ethics*. New York: Plenum Press.

Macklin, R. (1995). Maternal-fetal conflict II. In A. Goldworth, W. Silverman, D. Stevenson & F. Young (Eds.) *Ethics and perinatology*. New York: Oxford University Press.

March of Dimes. (2000). *March of Dimes research annual report: The promise of science—Investment in genetics*. White Plains, NY: Author.

March of Dimes. (2002a). *Preterm births, 1990-2000*. [Online]. Available: www.marchofdimes.com/aboutus/1531.asp

March of Dimes. (2002b). *Umbilical cord blood*. [Online]. Available: www.marchofdimes.com/aboutus/681_1160.asp

March of Dimes. (2003). *Cocaine use during pregnancy*. [Online]. Available: www.marchofdimes.com/professionals/681_1169.asp

Mathias, R. (1995). NIDA Survey provides first national data on drug use during pregnancy. *NIDA Notes: Women and Drug Abuse, 10*(1), 1-3. [Online]. Available: www.nida.nih.gov/NIDA_Notes/NNVol10N1/NIDASurvey.html

Meighan, M., Davis, M.W., Thomas, S.P. & Droppleman, P.G. (1999). Living with postpartum depression: The father's experience. *MCN, The American Journal of Maternal-Child Nursing, 24*(4), 202-208.

Melgar, C., Rosenfield, D., Rawlinson, K. & Greenberg, M. (1991). Perinatal outcome after multifetal reduction to twins compared with nonreduced multiple gestation. *Obstetrics and Gynecology, 78*(5), 763-766.

Meslin, E. (2000). Of clones, stem cells, and children: Issues and challenges in human research ethics. *Journal of Women's Health & Gender-Based Medicine, 9*(8), 831-841.

Meyer, A.W. (1939). *The rise of embryology*. Stanford, CA: Stanford University Press.

Mill, J.S. (1987). *Utilitarianism*. Buffalo, NY: Prometheus Books.

Miya, P., Pinch, W., Boardman, K., Keene, A., Spielman, M. & Harr, K. (1995). Ethical perceptions of parents and nurses in NICU: The case of baby Michael. *JOGNN, 24*(2), 125-130.

Moreno, J. (1987). Ethical and legal issues in the care of the impaired newborn. *Clinics in Perinatalogy, 14*(2), 345-359.

Muraskas, J., Marshall, P.A., Tomich, P., Myers, T.F., Gianopoulos, J.G. & Thomasma, D.C. (1999). Neonatal viability in the 1900s: Held hostage by technology. *Cambridge Quarterly of Healthcare Ethics, 8,* 160-172.

National Advisory Board on Ethics in Reproduction. (1994). Report on human cloning through embryo splitting: An amber light. *Kennedy Institute of Ethics Journal, 4*(3), 251-282.

National Bioethics Advisory Commission. (2001). *Ethical and policy issues in research involving human participants. Volume I: Report and Recommendations of the National Bioethics Advisory Commission*. Bethesda, MD: Author.

National Commission for the Protection of Human Subjects of Biomedical and Behavioral Research. (1979). *The Belmont Report: Ethical principles and guidelines for the protection of human subjects of research*. Washington, DC: Author.

National Institutes of Health. (2001). *Stem cells: Scientific progress and future research*. [Online.] Available: www.nih.gov/news/stemcell/scireport.htm

Newland, K. (1982). Infant mortality in socially vulnerable populations. *World Health Forum, 3*(3). 321-324.

Niska, K., Lia-Hoagberg, B. & Snyder, M. (1994). Parental concerns of Mexican-American first-time mothers and fathers. *Public Health Nursing, 14*(2), 111-117.

Norton, M., Merrill, J., Cooper, B., Kuller, J. & Clyman, R. (1993). Neonatal complications after the administration of indomethacin for preterm labor. *The New England Journal of Medicine, 329*(22), 1602-1607.

NOVA. (2001). *Eighteen ways to have a baby*. [Online.] Available: www.pbs.org/nova/transcripts/2811baby.html.

O'Keefe, M. (2001). *Nursing practice and the law: Avoiding malpractice and other legal risks*. Philadelphia: F.A. Davis Company.

Omery, A. (1989). Values, moral reasoning and ethics. *Nursing Clinics of North America, 24*(2), 499-508.

Patient Self-Determination Act of 1990. 42 U.C.S., Section 1396(a).

Pence, G.E. (2000). *Classical cases in medical ethics* (3rd ed.). Boston: McGraw Hill.

Phibbs, C., Bronstein, J., Buxton, E. & Phibbs, R. (1996). The effects of patient volume and level of care at the hospital of birth on neonatal morbidity. *JAMA, 276,* 1054-1059.

Phillips, C. (1997). *Mother-baby nursing.* Washington, DC: Association of Women's Health, Obstetrical and Neonatal Nurses.

Pinch, W. (2001). Cord blood banking: Ethical implications. *AJN, 101*(10), 55-59.

Pinelli, J. (2000). Effects of family coping and resources on family adjustment and parental stress in the acute phase of the NICU experience. *Neonatal Network, 19*(6), 27-37.

Plato. (1998). *The republic.* Oxford: Oxford University Press.

Pollack, H., Lantz, P. & Frohna, J. (2000). Maternal smoking and adverse birth outcomes among singletons and twins. *American Journal of Public Health, 90*(3), 395-400.

Porrelo, R., Burke, S. & Hendrix, M. (1991). Reduction of triplets and pregnancy outcome. *Obstetrics & Gynecology, 78*(3, Part 1), 335-339.

Press, A. (1984, July 2). Troubling test tube legacy. *Newsweek,* p. 54.

Promise of seven babies becomes ordeal for Frustaci family in 1985. (1997, November 21). *The Des Moines Register,* 8.

Rawls, J. (1999). *A theory of justice* (revised ed.). Cambridge, MA: Belnap Press/Harvard University Press.

Reed, B.G. (1987). Developing women-sensitive drug dependence treatment services: Why so difficult? *Journal of Psychoactive Drugs, 19,* 151-164.

Regan, D., Ehrlich, S. & Finnegan, L. (1987). Infants of drug addicts: At risk for child abuse, neglect and placement in foster care. *Neurotoxicology & Teratology, 9*(4), 315-319.

Resnick, M., Wattenberg, E. & Brewer, R. (1994). The fate of the non-marital child: A challenge to the health system. *Journal of Community Health, 19*(4), 285-301.

Rimmerman, A. & Sheran, H. (2001). The transition of Israeli men to fatherhood: A comparison between new fathers of pre-term/full-term infants. *Child & Family Social Work, 6*(3), 261-267.

Roe v. Wade. 410 U.S. 113 (1973).

Rumbold, G. (1999). *Ethics in nursing practice* (3rd ed.). London: Harcourt Brace and Company Limited.

Ryan, G.M. (1975). Toward improving the outcome of pregnancy: Recommendations for the regional development of perinatal services. *Obstetrics and Gynecology, 46,* 375-384.

Ryan, K. (1990). Erosion of the rights of pregnant women: In the interest of fetal well-being. Women's Health Issues, 1(1), 21-24.

Sachs, A. (1989, May 22). Here comes the pregnancy police: Mothers of drug-exposed infants face legal punishment. *Time*, p. 102.

Samuelsson, M., Rådestad, I. & Segesten, K. (2001). A waste of life: Fathers' experience of losing a child before birth. *Birth*, *28*(2), 124-30.

Scanzoni, J. & Marsiglio, W. (1993). New action theory and contemporary families. *Journal of Family Issues*, *14*(1), 105-132.

Savage, T.A. (1997). Ethical decision making for children. *Crit Care Nurs Clin North Am*, *9*(1), 97-105.

Schoendorf, K. & Kiely, J. (1992). Relationship of sudden infant death syndrome to maternal smoking during pregnancy. *Pediatrics*, *90*(6), 905-908.

Seay, J. (1996). *Health care as a human right under international law: An opportunity for new leadership.* Mill Valley, CA: Forum for Health Care Planning.

Selleck, C. & Redding, B. (1998). Knowledge and attitudes of registered nurses toward perinatal substance abuse. *Journal of Obstetric, Gynecologic & Neonatal Nursing*, *27*(1), 70-77.

Shiono, P. & Behrman, R. (1995). Low birthweight: Analysis and recommendations. *The Future of Children*, *5*(1), 4-18.

Snowden, F. (1985). Bioethical challenges at the dawn of life: An introduction. In C. Harris & F. Snowden (Eds.), *Bioethical Frontiers in Perinatal Intensive Care.* Natchitoches, LA: Northwestern University Press.

Soules, M. (2001). Human reproductive cloning: Not ready for prime time. *Fertility & Sterility*, *76*(2), 232-234.

Stainton, C., Murphy, B., Higgins, P.G., Neff, J.A., Nyberg, K. & Ritchie, J.A. (1999). The needs of postbirth parents: An international, multisite study. *Journal of Perinatal Education*, *8*(3), 21-29.

Stotland, N. (1990). Social change and women's reproductive health care. *Women's Health Issues*, *1*(1), 4-14.

Strong, C. (1991). Review: Court-ordered treatment in obstetrics. The ethical views and legal framework. *Obstetrics & Gynecology*, *78*(5 Part1), 861-868.

Strong, T.H. (2000). *Expecting trouble: The myth of prenatal care in America.* New York: New York University Press.

Sydnor-Greenberg, N. & Dokken, D. (2000). Family matters. Coping and caring in different ways: Understanding and meaningful involvement. *Pediatric Nursing*, *26*(2), 185-190.

Tanner, C., Benner, P., Chesla, C. & Gordon, D. (1993). The phenomenology of knowing the patient. *Image*, *25*, 273-280.

Teilhard de Chardin, P. (1976). *The phenomenon of man.* New York: Harper & Row.

Thompson, J.E. & Thompson, H.O. (1985). *Bioethical decision-making for nurses.* Norwalk, CT: Appleton-Century-Crofts.

Tiedje, L. (2000). Moral distress in perinatal nursing. *Journal of Perinatal and Neonatal Nursing, 14*(2), 36-43.

Tjaden, P. & Thoennes, N. (1998). Prevalence, incidence and consequences of violence against, women: Findings from the national violence against women survey. *Research in Brief.* Washington DC: U.S. Department of Justice.

Tomich, P. & Anderson, C. (1990). Analysis of a maternal transport service within a perinatal region. *American Journal of Perinatology, 7*(1), 13-17.

United Nations. (1959). *Preamble: Declaration of the rights of the child.* DOCA, 4354. New York: United Nations.

U.S. Bureau of the Census. (1991). *Census & you.* Washington, DC: U.S. Government Printing Office.

U.S. Department of Health, Education and Welfare (DHEW). (1979). *Healthy people: The Surgeon General's report on health promotion and disease prevention, 1979.* DHEW Publication No.79-55071. Washington DC: Author.

U.S. Department of Health and Human Services (DHHS). (1990). *Healthy people 2000: National health promotion and disease prevention objectives.* Boston: Jones and Bartlett.

U.S. Department of Health and Human Services (DHHS). (2000). *Healthy people, 2010.* Washington, DC: Author.

U.S. Department of Health and Human Services (DHHS). (2001). *Health United States, 2001.* Washington, DC: Author.

Van Zyl, L. & Van Kiekark, A. (2000). Interpretative perspectives and intentions in surrogate motherhood. *Journal of Medicine and Ethics, 26*(5), 404-409.

Vernon, J. (1998). Whatever happened to Baby Doe? *Neonatal Network, 17*(2), 73-74.

Vimpani, G. (1991). Resource allocation in contemporary pediatrics: The case against high technology. *Journal of Pediatric & Child Health, 27*(6), 354-359.

Walfisch, A., Hallak, M. & Mazor, M. (2001). Multiple courses of antenatal steroids: Risks and benefits. *Obstetrics & Gynecology, 98*(3), 491-497.

Wall, S. & Partridge, J. (1997). Death in the intensive care nursery: Physician practice of withdrawing and withholding life support. *Pediatrics, 99*(1), 64-70.

White, G. (1992). Understanding the ethical issues in infertility nursing practice. *NAACOG's Clinical Issues in Perinatal and Women's Health Nursing, 3*, 347-352.

REFERENCES

Wilkinson, J.M. (1987-1988). Moral distress in nursing practice: Experience and effect. *Nursing Forum, 23,* 16-29.

Wolf, S. (1996). *Feminism and bioethics: Beyond reproduction.* New York: Oxford University Press.

Woodhouse, L.D. (1992). Women with jagged edges: Voices from a culture of substance abuse. *Qualitative Health Research, 2*(3), 262-281.

Yeast, J.D., Poskin, M., Stockbauer, J.W. & Shaffer, S. (1998). Changing patterns in regionalization of perinatal care and the impact on neonatal mortality. American *Journal of Obstetrics & Gynecology, 178*(Pt. 1), 131-135.

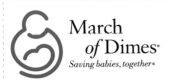

March *of* **Dimes**®
Saving babies, together®

March of Dimes
P.O. Box 932852
Atlanta, GA 31193-2852
Phone: 1-800-367-6630
Outside U.S.: 1-770-280-4115
Fax: 1-770-280-4116
Please use this form
when faxing orders.

Ship to:

Name _____

Company _____

Address _____

City _____ State _____ Zip _____

Daytime Phone (____) _____ Fax (____) _____

E-mail _____

Bill to: *(if different than ship to address)*

Name _____

Company _____

Address _____

City _____ State _____ Zip _____

Daytime Phone (____) _____ Fax (____) _____

E-mail _____

ITEM #	MODULE	QUANTITY	PRICE EACH	TOTAL
33-1437-01	Abuse During Pregnancy: A Protocol for Prevention and Intervention, 2nd Edition		$20	
33-1434-00	Adolescent Pregnancy, 2nd Edition		$20	
33-1610-01	The Art and Science of Labor Support		$20	
33-805-97	Assessment of Risk in the Term Newborn		$20	
33-720-00	Breastfeeding the Healthy Newborn: A Nursing Perspective		$20	
33-779-97	Breastfeeding the Infant with Special Needs		$20	
33-1656-02	Cultural Competence in the Care of Childbearing Families		$20	
33-1806-03	Diabetes in Pregnancy, 3rd Edition		$20	
33-1433-00	Discharge and Follow-Up of the High-Risk Preterm Infant		$20	
33-681-96	Easing the Transition from Hospital to Home		$20	
33-1520-01	Embryonic and Fetal Evaluation During Pregnancy		$20	
33-1828-03	Perinatal and Neonatal Ethics: Facing Contemporary Challenges		$20	
33-1751-02	Genetic Issues for Perinatal Nurses, 2nd Edition		$20	
33-676-00	Hemodynamic Monitoring of the Critically Ill Obstetric Patient		$20	
33-804-99	High-Risk Antepartal Home Care		$20	
33-900-98	High-Risk Pregnancy: Chronic Medical Conditions		$20	
33-891-97	Hypertensive Disorders of Pregnancy		$20	
33-1547-01	Loss and Grieving in Pregnancy and the First Year of Life: A Caring Resource for Nurses		$20	
33-675-00	The Mature Gravida: Pregnancy at Age 35 and Older		$20	
33-910-98	Nursing Assessment of the Pregnant Woman		$20	
33-808-97	Nursing Management of Multiple Birth Families		$20	
33-809-96	Obstetrical Emergencies for the Perinatal Nurse		$20	
33-1828-03	Perinatal and Neonatal Ethics: Facing Contemporary Challenges		$20	
33-1216-99	Perinatal Impact of Alcohol, Tobacco and Other Drugs		$20	
33-1680-00	Preconception Health Promotion: A Focus on Women's Wellness		$20	
33-1451-00	Pregnancy: Psychosocial Perspectives, 3rd Edition		$20	
33-806-99	The Premature Infant: Nursing Assessment and Management		$20	
33-1805-03	Preterm Labor: Prevention and Nursing Management, 3rd Edition		$20	
33-678-00	Window of Opportunity: Interviewing by the Perinatal Nurse		$20	
33-1755-02	Package 1: Perinatal Care of the Low-Risk Woman		$85	
33-1528-01	Package 2: Neonatal Care		$85	
33-1756-02	Package 3: Perinatal Care of the High-Risk Woman		$187	
33-1757-02	Package 4: Psychosocial Issues		$119	
			SUBTOTAL	
			SALES TAX *(CA only)*	
			SHIPPING *(see back side of form)*	
			TOTAL	

Method of Payment: *(Payment must accompany orders from individuals.)*

☐ Check – Payable to March of Dimes   ☐ Visa   ☐ American Express   ☐ Master Card   ☐ Discover

☐ Purchase Order # _____   Account Number _____   Exp. Date _____

Chapter Code _____   Signature _____

All orders less than $50.00 must be prepaid. Prices are subject to change without notice.

33-1828-03

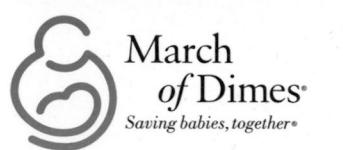

March of Dimes
P.O. Box 932852
Atlanta, GA 31193-2852

Phone: 1-800-367-6630
Outside U.S.: 1-770-280-4115
Fax: 1-770-280-4116
Please use this form
when faxing orders.

Standard Shipping and Handling Charges

ORDER TOTAL	S&H CHARGE
$1 – $75	$5.95
$76 – $499	17%
$500 – $999	15%
Over $1,000	12%

Call 1-800-367-6630 for rates for overnight, 2nd-day and same-day delivery and foreign shipments.

All orders outside the U.S. must be prepaid.

Please allow 2 weeks for delivery from the date we receive your order.

← Fold Line

PLACE
POSTAGE
HERE

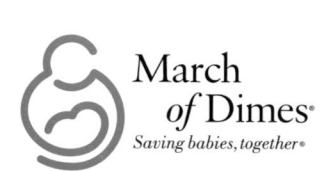

March of Dimes
P.O. Box 932852
Atlanta, GA 31193-2852

Fold Line →

15% savings over individual module purchase

Pre-Packaged Nursing Modules

Designed to meet the ongoing educational needs of nurses working in maternal and infant health

Package 1: Perinatal Care of the Low-Risk Woman
Item # 33-1755-02 $85

The Art & Science of Labor Support
Easing the Transition from Hospital to Home
Nursing Assessment of the Pregnant Woman
Preconception Health Promotion
Window of Opportunity: Interviewing by the
  Perinatal Nurse

Package 2: Neonatal Care
Item # 33-1528-01 $85

Assessment of Risk in the Term Newborn
Breastfeeding the Healthy Newborn
Breastfeeding the Infant with Special Needs
Discharge and Follow-Up of the High-Risk Preterm Infant
The Premature Infant: Nursing Assessment and
  Management

Package 3: Perinatal Care of the High-Risk Woman
Item # 33-1756-02 $187

Diabetes in Pregnancy, 3rd Edition
Embryonic & Fetal Evaluation During Pregnancy
Genetic Issues for Perinatal Nurses, 2nd Edition
Hemodynamic Monitoring of the Critically Ill Obstetric
  Patient
High-Risk Antepartal Home Care
High-Risk Pregnancy: Chronic Medical Conditions
Hypertensive Disorders of Pregnancy
The Mature Gravida: Pregnancy at Age 35 and Older
Nursing Management of Multiple Birth Families
Obstetrical Emergencies for the Perinatal Nurse
Preterm Labor: Prevention and Nursing Management,
  3rd Edition

Package 4: Psychosocial Issues
Item # 33-1757-02 $119

Abuse During Pregnancy, 2nd Edition
Adolescent Pregnancy, 2nd Edition
Cultural Competence in the Care of Childbearing
  Families
Loss & Grieving in Pregnancy and the First Year
  of Life
Perinatal and Neonatal Ethics: Facing Contemporary
  Challenges
Perinatal Impact of Alcohol, Tobacco and Other Drugs
Pregnancy: Psychosocial Perspectives, 3rd Edition

Perinatal and Neonatal Ethics: Facing Contemporary Challenges

Please remove and complete the evaluation, fold and staple it to reveal the postage-paid portion, and post it in a U.S. mailbox. (Note: Independent study takers can submit the evaluation with their tests for grading; group study participants can give the evaluation to their facilitator.) Thank you in advance for your time. Your responses are important to us as we plan additional continuing education activities.

1. **State(s) in which you currently practice**

   _____

2. **Professional identification** *(Check all that apply.)*
   - ☐ Registered nurse
   - ☐ Nurse practitioner
   - ☐ Clinical nurse specialist
   - ☐ Certified nurse-midwife
   - ☐ Childbirth educator
   - ☐ Nursing student
   - ☐ Other *(Please identify.)* _____

3. **Educational degree(s)** *(Check all that apply.)*
   - ☐ Diploma nurse
   - ☐ Associate degree
   - ☐ Baccalaureate in nursing
   - ☐ Baccalaureate in other field *(Please identify.)*
     _____
   - ☐ Master's in nursing
   - ☐ Master's in other field *(Please identify.)*
     _____
   - ☐ Doctorate in nursing
   - ☐ Doctorate in other field *(Please identify.)*
     _____

4. **Area(s) of certification**

   _____

5. **Current employment setting**
   - ☐ Hospital
   - ☐ Clinic
   - ☐ Private practice
   - ☐ Other *(Please identify.)* _____

6. **Type of work**
   - ☐ Administration
   - ☐ Education—academic/clinical
   - ☐ Clinical practice
   - ☐ Public health
   - ☐ Other *(Please identify.)* _____

7. **Length of time employed in the health care field**
   - ☐ <1 year
   - ☐ 1 to 2 years
   - ☐ 2 to 10 years
   - ☐ 10 to 20 years
   - ☐ >20 years

8. **How did you find out about this module?**
   - ☐ March of Dimes chapter
   - ☐ March of Dimes National Office
   - ☐ March of Dimes Web site
   - ☐ Conference
   - ☐ Place of employment
   - ☐ Peer/Colleague recommendation
   - ☐ Other *(Please identify.)* _____
     _____

9. **Have you used other nursing modules?**
   - ☐ Yes   ☐ No   ☐ Unsure

10. **If you are a prior module user, how many modules have you used?** _____

11. **If you are a prior module user, when was the last time you used a module?**
    - ☐ <1 month ago
    - ☐ 1 month to 1 year ago
    - ☐ 1 to 2 years ago
    - ☐ >2 years ago

12. **How did you use this module?**
    - ☐ Independent study for continuing education credit
    - ☐ Group study for continuing education credit
    - ☐ As a learning tool without continuing education credit
    - ☐ Other *(Please identify.)* _____
      _____

13. **Time required to read the module and complete the independent study test, if applicable**

    ____hours   ____minutes   ☐ Not applicable

14. **Time required to read the module and participate in the facilitated group study, if applicable**

    ____hours   ____minutes   ☐ Not applicable

Rate each of the following:

	Excellent	Very Good	Good	Fair	Poor	N/A
15. Cognitive objectives	____	____	____	____	____	____
16. Relationship of cognitive objectives to the overall purpose of the module	____	____	____	____	____	____
17. Expected practice outcomes	____	____	____	____	____	____
18. Key concepts	____	____	____	____	____	____
19. Content	____	____	____	____	____	____
20. Clinical application	____	____	____	____	____	____
21. Group discussion items	____	____	____	____	____	____
22. References	____	____	____	____	____	____
23. Supplementary materials	____	____	____	____	____	____
24. Overall quality of the module	____	____	____	____	____	____
25. Effectiveness of the module as teaching/learning material	____	____	____	____	____	____
26. Effectiveness of module as a means to increase awareness of the issue/topic	____	____	____	____	____	____

(Continued on other side)

27. **Which may change as a result of completing this module?**
    - ☐ Your attitude
    - ☐ Your knowledge base
    - ☐ Your skill level
    - ☐ Other *(Please identify.)* _____

28. **How might your use of the nursing process be affected by the module?**
    - ☐ Improved data collection
    - ☐ Improved client assessment
    - ☐ Improved accuracy in nursing diagnoses
    - ☐ Improved discharge planning
    - ☐ Improved (more appropriate) nursing interventions
    - ☐ Improved evaluation of nursing care
    - ☐ Other *(Please identify.)* _____

29. **Would you recommend this module to a colleague?**
    - ☐ Yes   ☐ No   ☐ Unsure

30. **How can the module be improved?**
    _____
    _____
    _____

31. **Suggestions for future module topics**
    _____
    _____
    _____

32. **Other comments**
    _____
    _____
    _____

← Fold Line

BUSINESS REPLY MAIL
FIRST CLASS • PERMIT NO. 2000 • WHITE PLAINS, NY

POSTAGE WILL BE PAID BY ADDRESSEE

March of Dimes Birth Defects Foundation
Education Services
1275 Mamaroneck Avenue
White Plains, NY 10602-9989

NO POSTAGE
NECESSARY IF
MAILED
IN THE
UNITED STATES

Fold Line →

1. **Number of participants attending the study**
   _____

2. **Location of the study**
   _____

3. **Date of the study**
   _____

4. **Length time for the study**
   _____

5. **When was the study held?**
   - ☐ During compensated on-duty time
   - ☐ As an overtime (paid) activity
   - ☐ On noncompensated time
   - ☐ Other *(Please identify.)* _____

6. **Reasons for the group study** *(Check all that apply.)*
   - ☐ To offer/obtain continuing education credit
   - ☐ To cross-train staff
   - ☐ To enhance clinical skills
   - ☐ Other *(Please identify.)* _____
   _____

7. **Did you offer/obtain continuing education credit for the module from the March of Dimes?**
   - ☐ Yes   ☐ No

8. **How could the group study process be improved?**
   _____
   _____

Books

Beauchamp, T.L. & Childress, J.F. (1994). *Principles of biomedical ethics* (4th. Ed.). New York: Oxford University Press.

Burkhart, M.A. & Nathaniel, A.K. (1998). *Ethics and issues in contemporary nursing.* Clifton Park, NY: Delmar Publishers.

Fry, S.T. & Veatch, R.M. (2000). *Case studies in nursing ethics* (2nd Ed.). Boston: Jones & Bartlet Publishers.

Hall, J.K. (1996). *Nursing ethics and law.* Philadelphia: W.B. Saunders.

Jonsen, A.R., Seigler, M. & Winslade, W.J. (1998). *Clinical ethics* (4th Ed.). New York: Macmillan Publishers.

Lantos, J. (2001). *The Lazarus case.* Baltimore, MD: Johns Hopkins University Press.

Lewis, M.A. & Tamparo, C.D. (1998). *Medical law, ethics and bioethics for ambulatory care* (4th Ed.). Philadelphia: F.A. Davis Company.

Loewy, E.H. (1996). *Textbook of healthcare ethics.* New York: Plenum Press.

Parens, E. & Asch, A. (Eds.). (2000). *Prenatal testing and disability rights.* Hastings Center Studies in Ethics. Washington DC: Georgetown University Press.

Pence, G.E. (2000). *Classic cases in medical ethics* (3rd Ed.). Boston: McGraw Hill.

Singer, P. (1994). *Rethinking life and death.* New York: St. Martin's Press.

Web sites

American Nurses Association (ANA)
nursingworld.com

ANA position statement index
nursingworld.org/readroom/position/index.htm

ANA position statement: *Ethics and Human Rights*
nursingworld.org/readroom/position/ethics/etethr.htm

The Center for Ethics and Human Rights
nursingworld.org/ethics/elinks.htm

American Hospital Association (AHA)
aha.org

The Patient's Bill of Rights
hospitalconnect.com/aha/about/pbillofrights.html

United Nations (UN)
un.org

Universal Declaration of Human Rights
un.org/overview/rights.htm

Professional Bioethics Organizations

American Society for Bioethics and Humanities (ASBH)
asbh.org

American Society for Law, Medicine and Ethics (ASLME)
aslme.org

Association of Women's Health, Obstetrical and Neonatal Nursing (AWHONN)
awhonn.org

Canadian Bioethics Society
bioethics.ca/english/index.html

Georgetown University
georgetown.edu

   The Kennedy Institute of Ethics
   georgetown.edu/research/kie

   Bioethics Information Retrieval Project
   georgetown.edu/research/nrcbl/ir/bioline.htm

National Catholic Bioethics Center
ncbcenter.org

Nursing Ethics at Boston College School of Nursing
bc.edu/nursing/ethics

Public Responsibility in Medicine and Research (PRIMR)
primr.org

The Society for Medical Decision Making (SMDM)
smdm.org

American Nurses' Association Code of Ethics for Nurses with Interpretive Statements

1. The nurse, in all professional relationships, practices with compassion and respect for the inherent dignity, worth and uniqueness of every individual, unrestricted by considerations of social or economic status, personal attributes, or the nature of health problems.

1.1 Respect for human dignity

A fundamental principle that underlies all nursing practice is respect for the inherent worth, dignity, and human rights of every individual. Nurses take into account the needs and values of all persons in all professional relationships.

1.2 Relationships to patients

The need for health care is universal, transcending all individual differences. The nurse establishes relationships and delivers nursing services with respect for human needs and values, and without prejudice. An individual's lifestyle, value system and religious beliefs should be considered in planning health care with and for each patient. Such consideration does not suggest that the nurse necessarily agrees with or condones certain individual choices, but that the nurse respects the patient as a person.

1.3 The nature of health problems

The nurse respects the worth, dignity and rights of all human beings irrespective of the nature of the health problem. The worth of the person is not affected by disease, disability, functional status, or proximity to death. This respect extends to all who require the services of the nurse for the promotion of health, the prevention of illness, the restoration of health, the alleviation of suffering, and the provision of supportive care to those who are dying.

The measures nurses take to care for the patient enable the patient to live with as much physical, emotional, social, and spiritual well-being as possible. Nursing care aims to maximize the values that the patient has treasured in life and extends supportive care to the family and significant others. Nursing care is directed toward meeting the comprehensive needs of patients and their families across the continuum of care. This is particularly vital in the care of patients and their families at the end of life to prevent and relieve the cascade of symptoms and suffering that are commonly associated with dying.

Nurses are leaders and vigilant advocates for the delivery of dignified and humane care. Nurses actively participate in assessing and assuring the responsible and appropriate use of interventions in order to minimize unwarranted or unwanted treatment and patient suffering. The acceptability and importance of carefully considered decisions regarding resuscitation status, withholding and withdrawing life-sustaining therapies, forgoing medically provided nutrition and hydration, aggressive pain and symptom management and advance directives are increasingly evident. The nurse should provide interventions to relieve pain and other symptoms in the dying patient even when those interventions entail risks of hastening death. However, nurses may not act with the sole intent of ending a patient's life even though such action may be motivated by compassion, respect for patient autonomy and quality of life considerations. Nurses have invaluable experience, knowledge, and insight into care at the end of life and should be actively involved in related research, education, practice, and policy development.

1.4 The right to self-determination
Respect for human dignity requires the recognition of specific patient rights, particularly, the right of self-determination. Self-determination, also known as autonomy, is the philosophical basis for informed consent in health care. Patients have the moral and legal right to determine what will be done with their own person; to be given accurate, complete, and understandable information in a manner that facilitates an informed judgment; to be assisted with weighing the benefits, burdens, and available options in their treatment, including the choice of no treatment; to accept, refuse, or terminate treatment without deceit, undue influence, duress, coercion, or penalty; and to be given necessary support throughout the decision-making and treatment process. Such support would include the opportunity to make decisions with family and significant others and the provision of advice and support from knowledgeable nurses and other health professionals. Patients should be involved in planning their own health care to the extent they are able and choose to participate.

Each nurse has an obligation to be knowledgeable about the moral and legal rights of all patients to self-determination. The nurse preserves, protects, and supports those interests by assessing the patient's comprehension of both the information presented and the implications of decisions. In situations in which the patient lacks the capacity to make a decision, a designated surrogate decision-maker should be consulted. The role of the surrogate is to make decisions as the patient would, based upon the patient's previously expressed wishes and known values. In the absence of a designated surrogate decision-maker, decisions should be made in the best interests of the patient, considering the patient's personal values to the extent that they are known. The nurse supports patient self-determination by participating in discussions with surrogates, providing guidance and referral to other resources as necessary, and identifying and addressing problems in the decision-making process. Support of autonomy in the broadest sense also includes recognition that people of some cultures place less weight on individualism and choose to defer to family or community values in decision-making. Respect not just for the specific decision but also for the patient's method of decision-making is consistent with the principle of autonomy.

Individuals are interdependent members of the community. The nurse recognizes that there are situations in which the right to individual self determination may be outweighed or limited by the rights, health and welfare of others, particularly in relation to public health considerations. Nonetheless, limitation of individual rights must always be considered a serious deviation from the standard of care, justified only when there are no less restrictive means available to preserve the rights of others and the demands of justice.

1.5 Relationships with colleagues and others
The principle of respect for persons extends to all individuals with whom the nurse interacts. The nurse maintains compassionate and caring relationships with colleagues and others with a commitment to the fair treatment of individuals, to

integrity-preserving compromise, and to resolving conflict. Nurses function in many roles, including direct care provider, administrator, educator, researcher, and consultant. In each of these roles, the nurse treats colleagues, employees, assistants, and students with respect and compassion. This standard of conduct precludes any and all prejudicial actions, any form of harassment or threatening behavior, or disregard for the effect of one's actions on others. The nurse values the distinctive contribution of individuals or groups, and collaborates to meet the shared goal of providing quality health services.

2. The nurse's primary commitment is to the patient, whether an individual, family, group or community.

2.1 Primacy of the patient's interests
The nurse's primary commitment is to the recipient of nursing and health care services—the patient—whether the recipient is an individual, a family, a group, or a community. Nursing holds a fundamental commitment to the uniqueness of the individual patient, therefore, any plan of care must reflect that uniqueness. The nurse strives to provide patients with opportunities to participate in planning care, assures that patients find the plans acceptable and supports the implementation of the plan. Addressing patient interests requires recognition of the patient's place in the family or other networks of relationship. When the patient's wishes are in conflict with others, the nurse seeks to help resolve the conflict. Where conflict persists, the nurse's commitment remains to the identified patient.

2.2 Conflict of interest for nurses
Nurses are frequently put in situations of conflict arising from competing loyalties in the workplace, including situations of conflicting expectations from patients, families, physicians, colleagues, and in many cases, health care organizations and health plans. Nurses must examine the conflicts arising between their own personal and professional values, the values and interests of others who are also responsible for patient care and health care decisions, as well as those of patients. Nurses strive to resolve such conflicts in ways that ensure patient safety, guard the patient's best interests and preserve the professional integrity of the nurse.

Situations created by changes in health care financing and delivery systems, such as incentive systems to decrease spending, pose new possibilities of conflict between economic self-interest and professional integrity. The use of bonuses, sanctions, and incentives tied to financial targets are examples of features of health care systems that may present such conflict. Conflicts of interest may arise in any domain of nursing activity including clinical practice, administration, education, or research. Advanced practice nurses who bill directly for services and nursing executives with budgetary responsibilities must be especially cognizant of the potential for conflicts of interest. Nurses should disclose to all relevant parties (e.g., patients, employers, colleagues) any perceived or actual conflict of interest and in some situations should withdraw from further participation. Nurses in all roles must seek to ensure that employment arrangements are just and fair and do not create an unreasonable conflict between patient care and direct personal gain.

2.3 Collaboration

Collaboration is not just cooperation, but it is the concerted effort of individuals and groups to attain a shared goal. In health care, that goal is to address the health needs of the patient and the public. The complexity of health care delivery systems requires a multi-disciplinary approach to the delivery of services that has the strong support and active participation of all the health professions. Within this context, nursing's unique contribution, scope of practice, and relationship with other health professions needs to be clearly articulated, represented, and preserved. By its very nature, collaboration requires mutual trust, recognition, and respect among the health care team, shared decision-making about patient care, and open dialogue among all parties who have an interest in and a concern for health outcomes. Nurses should work to assure that the relevant parties are involved and have a voice in decision-making about patient care issues. Nurses should see that the questions that need to be addressed are asked and that the information needed for informed decision-making is available and provided. Nurses should actively promote the collaborative multi-disciplinary planning required to ensure the availability and accessibility of quality health services to all persons who have needs for health care.

Intra-professional collaboration within nursing is fundamental to effectively addressing the health needs of patients and the public. Nurses engaged in non-clinical roles, such as administration or research, while not providing direct care, nonetheless are collaborating in the provision of care through their influence and direction of those who do. Effective nursing care is accomplished through the interdependence of nurses in differing roles—those who teach the needed skills, set standards, manage the environment of care, or expand the boundaries of knowledge used by the profession. In this sense, nurses in all roles share a responsibility for the outcomes of nursing care.

2.4 Professional boundaries

When acting within one's role as a professional, the nurse recognizes and maintains boundaries that establish appropriate limits to relationships. While the nature of nursing work has an inherently personal component, nurse-patient relationships and nurse-colleague relationships have, as their foundation, the purpose of preventing illness, alleviating suffering, and protecting, promoting, and restoring the health of patients. In this way, nurse-patient and nurse-colleague relationships differ from those that are purely personal and unstructured, such as friendship. The intimate nature of nursing care, the involvement of nurses in important and sometimes highly stressful life events, and the mutual dependence of colleagues working in close concert all present the potential for blurring of limits to professional relationships. Maintaining authenticity and expressing oneself as an individual, while remaining within the bounds established by the purpose of the relationship, can be especially difficult in prolonged or long-term relationships. In all encounters, nurses are responsible for retaining their professional boundaries. When those professional boundaries are jeopardized, the nurse should seek assistance from peers or supervisors or take appropriate steps to remove her/himself from the situation.

3. The nurse promotes, advocates for, and strives to protect the health, safety, and rights of the patient.

3.1 Privacy

The nurse safeguards the patient's right to privacy. The need for health care does not justiFy unwanted intrusion into the patient's life. The nurse advocates for an environment that provides for sufficient physical privacy, including auditory privacy for discussions of a personal nature and policies and practices that protect the confidentiality of information.

3.2 Confidentiality

Associated with the right to privacy, the nurse has a duty to maintain confidentiality of all patient information. The patient's well-being could be jeopardized and the fundamental trust between patient and nurse destroyed by unnecessary access to data or by the inappropriate disclosure of identifiable patient information. The rights, well-being, and safety of the individual patient should be the primary factors in arriving at any professional judgment concerning the disposition of confidential information received from or about the patient, whether oral, written or electronic. The standard of nursing practice and the nurse's responsibility to provide quality care require that relevant data be shared with those members of the health care team who have a need to know. Only information pertinent to a patient's treatment and welfare is disclosed, and only to those directly involved with the patient's care. Duties of confidentiality, however, are not absolute and may need to be modified in order to protect the patient, other innocent parties, and in circumstances of mandatory disclosure for public health reasons.

Information used for purposes of peer review, third-party payments, and other quality improvement or risk management mechanisms may be disclosed only under defined policies, mandates, or protocols. These written guidelines must assure that the rights, well-being, and safety of the patient are protected. In general, only that information directly relevant to a task or specific responsibility should be disclosed. When using electronic communications, special effort should be made to maintain data security.

3.3 Protection of participants in research

Stemming from the right to self-determination, each individual has the right to choose whether or not to participate in research. It is imperative that the patient or legally authorized surrogate receive sufficient information that is material to an informed decision, to comprehend that information, and to know how to discontinue participation in research without penalty. Necessary information to achieve an adequately informed consent includes the nature of participation, potential harms and benefits, and available alternatives to taking part in the research. Additionally, the patient should be informed of how the data will be protected. The patient has the right to refuse to participate in research or to withdraw at any time without fear of adverse consequences or reprisal.

Research should be conducted and directed only by qualified persons. Prior to implementation, all research should be approved by a qualified review board to ensure patient protection and the ethical integrity of the research. Nurses should be cognizant of the special concerns raised by research involving vulnerable groups, including children, prisoners, students, the elderly, and the poor. The nurse who participates in research in any capacity should be fully informed about both the subject's and the nurse's rights and obligations in the particular research study and in research in general. Nurses have the duty to question and, if necessary, to report and to refuse to participate in research they deem morally objectionable.

3.4 Standards and review mechanisms

Nursing is responsible and accountable for assuring that only those individuals who have demonstrated the knowledge, skill, practice experiences, commitment, and integrity essential to professional practice are allowed to enter into and continue to practice within the profession. Nurse educators have a responsibility to ensure that basic competencies are achieved and to promote a commitment to professional practice prior to entry of an individual into practice. Nurse administrators are responsible for assuring that the knowledge and skills of each nurse in the workplace are assessed prior to the assignment of responsibilities requiring preparation beyond basic academic programs.

The nurse has a responsibility to implement and maintain standards of professional nursing practice. The nurse should participate in planning, establishing, implementing, and evaluating review mechanisms designed to safeguard patients and nurses, such as peer review processes or committees, credentialing processes, quality improvement initiatives, and ethics committees. Nurse administrators must ensure that nurses have access to and inclusion on institutional ethics committees. Nurses must bring forward difficult issues related to patient care and/or institutional constraints upon ethical practice for discussion and review. The nurse acts to promote inclusion of appropriate others in all deliberations related to patient care.

Nurses should also be active participants in the development of policies and review mechanisms designed to promote patient safety, reduce the likelihood of errors, and address both environmental system factors and human factors that present increased risk to patients. In addition, when errors do occur, nurses are expected to follow institutional guidelines in reporting errors committed or observed to the appropriate supervisory personnel and for assuring responsible disclosure of errors to patients. Under no circumstances should the nurse participate in, or condone through silence, either an attempt to hide an error or a punitive response that serves only to fix blame rather than correct the conditions that led to the error.

3.5 Acting on questionable practice

The nurse's primary commitment is to the health, well-being, and safety of the patient across the life span and in all settings in which health care needs are addressed. As an advocate for the patient, the nurse must be alert to and take appropriate action regarding any instances of incompetent, unethical, illegal, or impaired practice by any member of the health care team or the health care system or any action on the part of others that places the rights or best interests of the patient in jeopardy. To function effectively in this role, nurses must be knowledgeable about the *Code of Ethics*, standards of practice of the profession, relevant federal, state and local laws and regulations, and the employing organization's policies and procedures.

When the nurse is aware of inappropriate or questionable practice in the provision or denial of health care, concern should be expressed to the person carrying out the questionable practice. Attention should be called to the possible detrimental affect upon the patient's well-being or best interests as well as the integrity of nursing practice. When factors in the health care delivery system or health care organization threaten the welfare of the patient, similar action should be directed to the responsible administrator. If indicated, the problem should be reported to an appropriate higher authority within the institution or agency, or to an appropriate external authority.

There should be established processes for reporting and handling incompetent, unethical, illegal, or impaired practice within the employment setting so that such reporting can go through official channels, thereby reducing the risk of reprisal against the reporting nurse. All nurses have a responsibility to assist those who identify potentially questionable practice. State nurses associations should be prepared to provide assistance and support in the development and evaluation of such processes and reporting procedures. When incompetent, unethical, illegal, or impaired practice is not corrected within the employment setting and continues to jeopardize patient well-being and safety, the problem should be reported to other appropriate authorities such as practice committees of the pertinent professional organizations, the legally constituted bodies concerned with licensing of specific categories of health workers and professional practitioners, or the regulatory agencies concerned with evaluating standards or practice. Some situations may warrant the concern and involvement of all such groups. Accurate reporting and factual documentation, and not merely opinion, undergird all such responsible actions. When a nurse chooses to engage in the act of responsible reporting about situations that are perceived as unethical, incompetent, illegal, or impaired, the professional organization has a responsibility to provide the nurse with support and assistance and to protect the practice of those nurses who choose to voice their concerns. Reporting unethical, illegal, incompetent, or impaired practices, even when done appropriately, may present substantial risks to the nurse; nevertheless, such risks do not eliminate the obligation to address serious threats to patient safety.

3.6 Addressing impaired practice

Nurses must be vigilant to protect the patient, the public, and the profession from potential harm when a colleague's practice, in any setting, appears to be impaired. The nurse extends compassion and caring to colleagues who are in recovery from illness or when illness interferes with job performance. In a situation where a nurse suspects another's practice may be impaired, the nurse's duty is to take action designed both to protect patients and to assure that the impaired individual receives assistance in regaining optimal function. Such action should usually begin with consulting supervisory personnel and may also include confronting the individual in a supportive manner and with the assistance of others or helping the individual to access appropriate resources. Nurses are encouraged to follow guidelines outlined by the profession and policies of the employing organization to assist colleagues whose job performance may be adversely affected by mental or physical illness or by personal circumstances. Nurses in all roles should advocate for colleagues whose job performance may be impaired to ensure that they receive appropriate assistance, treatment and access to fair institutional and legal processes. This includes supporting the return to practice of the individual who has sought assistance and is ready to resume professional duties.

If impaired practice poses a threat or danger to self or others, regardless of whether the individual has sought help, the nurse must take action to report the individual to persons authorized to address the problem. Nurses who advocate for others whose job performance creates a risk for harm should be protected from negative consequences. Advocacy may be a difficult process and the nurse is advised to follow workplace policies. If workplace policies do not exist or are inappropriate—that is, they deny the nurse in question access to due legal process or demand resignation—the reporting nurse may obtain guidance from the professional association, state peer assistance programs, employee assistance program or a similar resource.

4. The nurse is responsible and accountable for individual nursing practice and determines the appropriate delegation of tasks consistent with the nurse's obligation to provide optimum patient care.

4.1 Acceptance of accountability and responsibility

Individual registered nurses bear primary responsibility for the nursing care that their patients receive and are individually accountable for their own practice. Nursing practice includes direct care activities, acts of delegation, and other responsibilities such as teaching, research, and administration. In each instance, the nurse retains accountability and responsibility for the quality of practice and for conformity with standards of care.

Nurses are faced with decisions in the context of the increased complexity and changing patterns in the delivery of health care. As the scope of nursing practice changes, the nurse must exercise judgment in accepting responsibilities, seeking consultation, and assigning activities to others who carry out nursing care. For example, some advanced practice nurses have the authority to issue prescription and treatment orders to be carried out by other nurses. These acts are not acts of delegation. Both the advanced practice nurse issuing the order and the nurse accepting the order are responsible for the judgments made and accountable for the actions taken.

4.2 Accountability for nursing judgment and action

Accountability means to be answerable to oneself and others for one's own actions. In order to be accountable, nurses act under a code of ethical conduct that is grounded in the moral principles of fidelity and respect for the dignity, worth, and self-determination of patients. Nurses are accountable for judgments made and actions taken in the course of nursing practice, irrespective of health care organizations' policies or providers' directives.

4.3 Responsibility for nursing judgment and action

Responsibility refers to the specific accountability or liability associated with the performance of duties of a particular role. Nurses accept or reject specific role demands based upon their education, knowledge, competence, and extent of experience. Nurses in administration, education, and research also have obligations to the recipients of nursing care. Although nurses in administration, education, and research have relationships with patients that are less direct, in assuming the responsibilities of a particular role, they share responsibility for the care provided by those whom they supervise and instruct. The nurse must not engage in practices prohibited by law or delegate activities to others that are prohibited by the practice acts of other health care providers.

Individual nurses are responsible for assessing their own competence. When the needs of the patient are beyond the qualifications and competencies of the nurse, consultation and collaboration must be sought from qualified nurses, other health professionals, or other appropriate sources. Educational resources should be sought by nurses and provided by institutions to maintain and advance the competence of nurses. Nurse educators act in collaboration with their students to assess the learning needs of the student, the effectiveness of the teaching program, the identification and utilization of appropriate resources, and the support needed for the learning process.

4.4 Delegation of nursing activities

Since the nurse is accountable for the quality of nursing care given to patients, nurses are accountable for the assignment of nursing responsibilities to other nurses and the delegation of nursing care activities to other health care workers. While delegation and assignment are used here in a generic moral sense, it is understood that individual states may have a particular legal definition of these terms.

The nurse must make reasonable efforts to assess individual competence when assigning selected components of nursing care to other health care workers. This assessment involves evaluating the knowledge, skills, and experience of the individual to whom the care is assigned, the complexity of the assigned tasks, and the health status of the patient. The nurse is also responsible for monitoring the activities of these individuals and evaluating the quality of the care provided. Nurses may not delegate responsibilities such as assessment and evaluation; they may delegate tasks. The nurse must not knowingly assign or delegate to any member of the nursing team a task for which that person is not prepared or qualified. Employer policies or directives do not relieve the nurse of responsibility for making judgments about the delegation and assignment of nursing care tasks.

Nurses functioning in management or administrative roles have a particular responsibility to provide an environment that supports and facilitates appropriate assignment and delegation. This includes providing appropriate orientation to staff, assisting less experienced nurses in developing necessary skills and competencies, and establishing policies and procedures that protect both the patient and nurse from the inappropriate assignment or delegation of nursing responsibilities, activities, or tasks.

Nurses functioning in educator or preceptor roles may have less direct relationships with patients. However, through assignment of nursing care activities to learners, they share responsibility and accountability for the care provided. It is imperative that the knowledge and skills of the learner be sufficient to provide the assigned nursing care and that appropriate supervision be provided to protect both the patient and the learner.

5. The nurse owes the same duties to self as to others, including the responsibility to preserve integrity and safety, to maintain competence, and to continue personal and professional growth.

5.1 Moral self-respect

Moral respect accords moral worth and dignity to all human beings irrespective of their personal attributes or life situation. Such respect extends to oneself as well; the same duties that we owe to others we owe to ourselves. Self-regarding duties refer to a realm of duties that primarily concern oneself and include professional growth and maintenance of competence, preservation of wholeness of character, and personal integrity.

5.2 Professional growth and maintenance of competence

Though it has consequences for others, maintenance of competence and ongoing professional growth involves the control of one's own conduct in a way that is primarily self-regarding. Competence affects one's self-respect, self-esteem, professional status, and the meaningfulness of work. In all nursing roles, evaluation of one's own performance, coupled with peer review, is a means by which nursing practice can be held to the highest standards. Each nurse is responsible for participating in the development of criteria for evaluation of practice and for using those criteria in peer and self-assessment.

Continual professional growth, particularly in knowledge and skill, requires a commitment to lifelong learning. Such learning includes, but is not limited to, continuing education, networking with professional colleagues, self-study, professional reading, certification, and seeking advanced degrees. Nurses are required to have knowledge relevant to the current scope and standards of nursing practice, changing issues, concerns, controversies, and ethics. Where the care required is outside the competencies of the individual nurse, consultation should be sought or the patient should be referred to others for appropriate care.

5.3 Wholeness of character

Nurses have both personal and professional identities that are neither entirely separate, nor entirely merged, but are integrated. In the process of becoming a professional, the nurse embraces the values of the profession, integrating them with personal values. Duties to self involve an authentic expression of one's own moral point-of-view in practice. Sound ethical decision-making requires the respectful and open exchange of views between and among all individuals with relevant interests. In a community of moral discourse, no one person's view should automatically take precedence over that of another. Thus the nurse has a responsibility to express moral perspectives, even when they differ from those of others, and even when they might not prevail.

This wholeness of character encompasses relationships with patients. In situations where the patient requests a personal opinion from the nurse, the nurse is generally free to express an informed personal opinion as long as this preserves the voluntariness of the patient and maintains appropriate professional and moral boundaries. It is essential to be aware of the potential for undue influence attached to the nurse's professional role. Assisting patients to clarify their own values in reaching informed decisions may be helpful in avoiding unintended persuasion. In situations where nurses' responsibilities include care for those whose personal attributes, condition, lifestyle, or situation is stigmatized by the community and are personally unacceptable, the nurse still renders respectful and skilled care.

5.4 Preservation of integrity

Integrity is an aspect of wholeness of character and is primarily a self-concern of the individual nurse. An economically constrained health care environment presents the nurse with particularly troubling threats to integrity. Threats to integrity may include a request to deceive a patient, to withhold information, or to falsify records, as well as verbal abuse from patients or coworkers. Threats to integrity also may include an expectation that the nurse will act in a way that is inconsistent with the values or ethics of the profession, or more specifically a request that is in direct violation of the *Code of Ethics*. Nurses have a duty to remain consistent with both their personal and professional values and to accept compromise only to the degree that it remains an integrity-preserving compromise. An integrity-preserving compromise does not jeopardize the dignity or well-being of the nurse or others. Integrity-preserving compromise can be difficult to achieve, but is more likely to be accomplished in situations where there is an open forum for moral discourse and an atmosphere of mutual respect and regard.

Where nurses are placed in situations of compromise that exceed acceptable moral limits or involve violations of the moral standards of the profession, whether in direct patient care or in any other forms of nursing practice, they may express their conscientious objection to participation. Where a particular treatment, intervention, activity, or practice is morally objectionable to the nurse, whether intrinsically so or because it is inappropriate for the specific patient, or where it may jeopardize both patients and nursing practice, the nurse is justified in refusing to participate on moral grounds. Such grounds exclude personal preference, prejudice, convenience, or arbitrariness. Conscientious objection may not insulate the nurse against formal or informal penalty. The nurse who decides not to take part on the grounds of conscientious objection must communicate this decision in appropriate ways. Whenever possible, such a refusal should be made known in advance and in time for alternate arrangements to be made for patient care. The nurse is obliged to provide for the patient's safety, to avoid patient abandonment, and to withdraw only when assured that alternative sources of nursing care are available to the patient.

Where patterns of institutional behavior or professional practice compromise the integrity of all its nurses, nurses should express their concern or conscientious objection collectively to the appropriate body or committee. In addition, they should express their concern, resist, and seek to bring about a change in those persistent activities or expectations in the practice setting that are morally objectionable to nurses and jeopardize either patient or nurse well-being.

6. The nurse participates in establishing, maintaining, and improving health care environments and conditions of employment conducive to the provision of quality health care and consistent with the values of the profession through individual and collective action.

6.1 Influence of the environment on moral virtues and values

Virtues are habits of character that predispose persons to meet their moral obligations; that is, to do what is right. Excellences are habits of character that predispose a person to do a particular job or task well. Virtues such as wisdom, honesty, and courage are habits or attributes of the morally good person. Excellences such as compassion, patience, and skill are habits of character of the morally good nurse. For the nurse, virtues and excellences are those habits that affirm and promote the values of human dignity, well-being, respect, health, independence, and other values central to nursing. Both virtues and excellences, as aspects of moral character, can be either nurtured by the environment in which the nurse practices or they can be diminished or thwarted. All nurses have a responsibility to create, maintain, and contribute to environments that support the growth of virtues and excellences and enable nurses to fulfill their ethical obligations.

6.2 Influence of the environment on ethical obligations

All nurses, regardless of role, have a responsibility to create, maintain, and contribute to environments of practice that support nurses in fulfilling their ethical obligations. Environments of practice include observable features, such as working conditions, and written policies and procedures setting out expectations for nurses, as well as less tangible characteristics such as informal peer norms. Organizational structures, role descriptions, health and safety initiatives, grievance mechanisms, ethics committees, compensation systems, and disciplinary procedures all contribute to environments that can either present barriers or foster ethical practice and professional fulfillment. Environments in which employees are provided fair hearing of grievances, are supported in practicing according to standards of care, and are justly treated allow for the realization of the values of the profession and are consistent with sound nursing practice.

6.3 Responsibility for the health care environment

The nurse is responsible for contributing to a moral environment that encourages respectful interactions with colleagues, support of peers, and identification of issues that need to be addressed. Nurse administrators have a particular responsibility to assure that employees are treated fairly and that nurses are involved in decisions related to their practice and working conditions. Acquiescing and accepting unsafe or inappropriate practices, even if the individual does not participate in the specific practice, is equivalent to condoning unsafe practice. Nurses should not remain employed in facilities that routinely violate patient rights or require nurses to severely and repeatedly compromise standards of practice or personal morality.

As with concerns about patient care, nurses should address concerns about the health care environment through appropriate channels. Organizational changes are difficult to accomplish and may require persistent efforts over time. Toward this end, nurses may participate in collective action such as collective bargaining or workplace advocacy, preferably through a professional association such as the state nurses association, in order to address the terms and conditions of employment. Agreements reached through such action must be consistent with the profession's standards of practice, the state law regulating practice, and the *Code of Ethics* for nursing. Conditions of employment must contribute to the moral environment, the provision of quality patient care, and the professional satisfaction for nurses.

The professional association also serves as an advocate for the nurse by seeking to secure just compensation and humane working conditions for nurses. To accomplish this, the professional association may engage in collective bargaining on behalf of nurses. While seeking to assure just economic and general welfare for nurses, collective bargaining, nonetheless, seeks to keep the interests of both nurses and patients in balance.

7. The nurse participates in the advancement of the profession through contributions to practice, education, administration, and knowledge development.

7.1 Advancing the profession through active involvement in nursing and in health care policy

Nurses should advance their profession by contributing in some way to the leadership, activities, and the viability of their professional organizations. Nurses can also advance the profession by serving in leadership or mentorship roles or on committees within their places of employment. Nurses who are self-employed can advance the profession by serving as role models for professional integrity. Nurses can also advance the profession through participation in civic activities related to health care or through local, state, national, or international initiatives. Nurse educators have a specific responsibility to enhance students' commitment to professional and civic values. Nurse administrators have a responsibility to foster an employment environment that facilitates nurses' ethical integrity and professionalism, and nurse researchers are responsible for active contribution to the body of knowledge supporting and advancing nursing practice.

7.2 Advancing the profession by developing, maintaining, and implementing professional standards in clinical, administrative, and educational practice

Standards and guidelines reflect the practice of nursing grounded in ethical commitments and a body of knowledge. Professional standards and guidelines for nurses must be developed by nurses and reflect nursing's responsibility to society. It is the responsibility of nurses to identify their own scope of practice as permitted by professional practice standards and guidelines, by state and federal laws, by relevant societal values, and by the *Code of Ethics*.

The nurse as administrator or manager must establish, maintain, and promote conditions of employment that enable nurses within that organization or community setting to practice in accord with accepted standards of nursing practice and provide a nursing and health care work environment that meets the standards and guidelines of nursing practice. Professional autonomy and self-regulation in the control of conditions of practice are necessary for implementing nursing standards and guidelines and assuring quality care for those whom nursing serves.

The nurse educator is responsible for promoting and maintaining optimum standards of both nursing education and of nursing practice in any settings where planned learning activities occur. Nurse educators must also ensure that only those students who possess the knowledge, skills, and competencies that are essential to nursing graduate from their nursing programs.

7.3 Advancing the profession through knowledge development, dissemination, and application to practice

The nursing profession should engage in scholarly inquiry to identify, evaluate, refine, and expand the body of knowledge that forms the foundation of its discipline and practice. In addition, nursing knowledge is derived from the sciences and from the humanities. Ongoing scholarly activities are essential to fulfilling a profession's obligations to society. All nurses working alone or in collaboration with others can participate in the advancement of the profession through the development, evaluation, dissemination, and application of knowledge in practice. However, an organizational climate and infrastructure conducive to scholarly inquiry must be valued and implemented for this to occur.

8. The nurse collaborates with other health professionals and the public in promoting community, national, and international efforts to meet health needs.

8.1 Health needs and concerns

The nursing profession is committed to promoting the health, welfare, and safety of all people. The nurse has a responsibility to be aware not only of specific health needs of individual patients but also of broader health concerns such as world hunger, environmental pollution, lack of access to health care, violation of human rights, and inequitable distribution of nursing and health care resources. The availability and accessibility of high quality health services to all people require both interdisciplinary planning and collaborative partnerships among health professionals and others at the community, national, and international levels.

8.2 Responsibilities to the public

Nurses, individually and collectively, have a responsibility to be knowledgeable about the health status of the community and existing threats to health and safety. Through support of and participation in community organizations and groups, the nurse assists in efforts to educate the public, facilitates informed choice, identifies conditions and circumstances that contribute to illness, injury and disease, fosters healthy lifestyles, and participates in institutional and legislative efforts to promote health and meet national health objectives. In addition, the nurse supports initiatives to address barriers to health, such as poverty, homelessness, unsafe living conditions, abuse and violence, and lack of access to health services.

The nurse also recognizes that health care is provided to culturally diverse populations in this country and in all parts of the world. In providing care, the nurse should avoid imposition of the nurse's own cultural values upon others. The nurse should affirm human dignity and show respect for the values and practices associated with different cultures and use approaches to care that reflect awareness and sensitivity.

9. The profession of nursing, as represented by associations and their members, is responsible for articulating nursing values, for maintaining the integrity of the profession and its practice, and for shaping social policy.

9.1 Assertion of values

It is the responsibility of a professional association to communicate and affirm the values of the profession to its members. It is essential that the professional organization encourages discourse that supports critical self-reflection and evaluation within the profession. The organization also communicates to the public the values that nursing considers central to social change that will enhance health.

9.2 The profession carries out its collective responsibility through professional associations

The nursing profession continues to develop ways to clarify nursing's accountability to society. The contract between the profession and society is made explicit through such mechanisms as (a) the *Code of Ethics for Nurses*, (b) the standards of nursing practice, (c) the ongoing development of nursing knowledge derived from nursing theory, scholarship, and research in order to guide nursing actions, (d) educational requirements for practice, (e) certification, and (f) mechanisms for evaluating the effectiveness of professional nursing actions.

9.3 Intraprofessional integrity

A professional association is responsible for expressing the values and ethics of the profession and also for encouraging the professional organization and its members to function in accord with those values and ethics. Thus, one of its fundamental responsibilities is to promote awareness of and adherence to the *Code of Ethics* and to critique the activities and ends of the professional association itself. Values and ethics influence the power structures of the association in guiding, correcting, and directing its activities. Legitimate concerns for the self-interest of the association and the profession are balanced by a commitment to the social goods that are sought. Through critical self-reflection and self-evaluation, associations must foster change within themselves, seeking to move the professional community toward its stated ideals.

9.4 Social reform

Nurses can work individually as citizens or collectively through political action to bring about social change. It is the responsibility of a professional nursing association to speak for nurses collectively in shaping and reshaping health care within our nation, specifically in areas of health care policy and legislation that affect accessibility, quality, and the cost of health care. Here, the professional association maintains vigilance and takes action to influence legislators, reimbursement agencies, nursing organizations, and other health professions. In these activities, health is understood as being broader than delivery and reimbursement systems, but extending to health-related sociocultural issues such as violation of human rights, homelessness, hunger, violence, and the stigma of illness.

From ANA, 2001; reprinted with permission

International Council of Nurses Position Statement: Rights of Children

The International Council of Nurses (ICN) endorses the Declaration of the Rights of the Child[1] and the Convention on the Rights of the Child[2] and supports efforts made by its member national nurses associations (NNAs) to promote the principles set forth in the Convention. More specifically, ICN supports:

- Protecting children from any form of abuse, sexual exploitation or child labor which damages their health and intellectual, physical, social and psychological development.

- Promoting family health and welfare so that the family unit is the place where children are wanted, protected and cared for to grow up in health and dignity.

- Lobbying for equitable distribution of goods and services so that all children have adequate nutrition, housing, education and health care and, promoting equal opportunities for education of female children, orphans and those of minority groups.

- Fostering the delivery of primary health care services with emphasis on the promotion of health, prevention of disease and disability.

- Enhancing protection and care for children with special needs such as orphans, abused or neglected and refugee children.

- Promoting the rights of the hospitalized child, including parental involvement in caring for the sick or institutionalized child or the child being cared for in the community.

Background
The UN Convention on the Rights of the Child affirms that:

Every child shall enjoy fundamental rights and freedoms regardless of race, colour, sex, language, religion, political or other opinion, national or social origin, property, birth or other status, whether of him/herself or of his/her family.

The child shall enjoy special protection and opportunity to develop physically, mentally, morally, spiritually and socially in conditions of freedom and dignity. The child shall be entitled from birth to a name and a nationality.

Special care and protection shall be provided for child and mother, including adequate pre-natal and post-natal care. The child shall have the right to adequate nutrition, housing, recreation and health services. The physically, mentally or socially handicapped child shall have special treatment, education and care.

The child shall grow up in an atmosphere of affection and of moral and material security. Wherever possible the child shall grow up in the care of and under the responsibility of parents and only in exceptional circumstances shall the infant be separated from the mother. Society and public authorities shall have the duty to extend particular care to children without family and those without adequate means of support.

There shall be equal opportunity to free and compulsory education, at least in elementary stages, which will promote the child's individual abilities, judgement and sense of moral and social responsibility. There shall be opportunity for play and recreation. In all circumstances the child shall be among the first to receive protection and relief.

The child shall be protected against all forms of neglect, cruelty and exploitation, and not be the subject of traffic in any form. There shall be an appropriate minimum age for employment, and no employment of children that would prejudice health or education or interfere with physical, mental or moral development.

The child shall be protected from practices, which cause racial, religious or any other form of discrimination, and be brought up in a spirit of tolerance, friendship among peoples, peace and consciousness of a responsibility for his/her fellow human beings.

---

[1]United Nations: The Declaration on the Rights of the Child. United Nations, adopted in 1959
[2]United Nations: The Convention on the Rights of the Child. United Nations, adopted November 20, 1989
Adopted in 1979
Revised in 2000
Available: www.icn.ch/pschildrights00.htm

International Council of Nurses Position Statement: Nurses and Human Rights

Human rights in health care involve both recipients and providers. The International Council of Nurses (ICN) views health care as a right of all individuals, regardless of financial, political, geographic, racial or religious considerations. This right includes the right to choose or decline care, including the right to accept or refuse treatment or nourishment; informed consent; confidentiality, and dignity, including the right to die with dignity.

Human Rights and the Nurse's Role

Nurses have an obligation to safeguard people's health rights at all times and in all places. This includes assuring that adequate care is provided within the resources available and in accordance with nursing ethics. As well, the nurse is obliged to ensure that patients receive appropriate information prior to consenting to treatment or procedures, including participation in research.

ICN advocates inclusion of human rights issues and the nurses' role in all levels of nursing education programs.

As professionals, nurses are accountable for their own actions in safeguarding human rights. National nurses' associations have a responsibility to participate in the development of health and social legislation related to patient rights.

Nurses' Rights

Nurses have the right to practice in accordance with the nursing legislation of the country in which they work and to adopt the ICN Code for Nurses or their own national ethical code. Nurses also have a right to practice in an environment that provides personal safety, freedom from abuse and violence, threats or intimidation.

National nurses' associations need to ensure an effective mechanism through which nurses can seek confidential advice, counsel, support and assistance in dealing with difficult human rights situations.

Background

Nurses deal with human rights issues daily, in all aspects of their professional role. Nurses may be pressured to apply their knowledge and skills in ways that are detrimental to patients and others. There is a need for increased vigilance, and a requirement to be well informed, about how new technology and experimentation can violate human rights. Furthermore nurses are increasingly facing complex human rights issues, arising from conflict situations within jurisdictions, political upheaval and wars. The application of human rights protection should emphasize vulnerable groups such as women, children, elderly, refugees and stigmatized groups.

ICN has developed Health and Human Rights fact sheet addressing the major areas where human rights impacts on the health of populations, including public health, health care reform, access to care and gender perspectives.

ICN endorses the Universal Declaration of Human rights, adopted in 1948.[1]

---

[1]Universal Declaration of Human rights (1948), New York: United Nations
Adopted in 1998
(Replaces previous ICN Position: *The Nurse's Role in Safeguarding Human Rights*, adopted 1983, updated 1993)
Available: http://www.icn.ch/pshumrights.htm

Figure 4. Laganá-Duderstadt Deontological Ethical Model

Step 1. Describe the ethical dilemma.

_____

_____

_____

_____

_____

Step 2. Identify alternative solutions.

_____

_____

_____

_____

_____

_____

_____

_____

_____

_____

3. Identify ethical principles.

_____

_____

_____

_____

_____

_____

_____

_____

**Step 4.
Analyze alternatives.**

Compare solutions
with principles.

One alternative
consistent with
rules or principles

↓

One right action

Alternative consistent
withone rule or principle
conflicts with another

↓

Appeal to higher-level
principle to solve conflict

Step 5. Take action.

_____

_____

_____

_____

_____

Adapted from Brody, 1981

Figure 5. Laganá-Duderstadt Utilitarian Ethical Model

Step 1. Identify the ethical dilemma.

_____
_____
_____
_____
_____

Step 2. Define possible actions.

_____
_____
_____
_____

Step 3. Consider consequences of each possible action.

_____
_____
_____
_____

Step 4. Identify those affected by the decision.

_____
_____
_____
_____

Step 5. Determine the degree of happiness for each affected party.

_____
_____
_____
_____

Step 6. Compare happiness scores.

_____
_____
_____

Adapted from Brody, 1981

APPENDIX 6

Figure 6. Laganá-Duderstadt Ethical Model of Caring

Step 1. State the ethical dilemma.

Step 2. Describe the context.

Step 3. Identify personal relationships.

Step 4. Analyze the power structure.

Step 5. Assess degree of informed consent.

Step 6. Identify significant values.

Step 7. Make a decision.